D0773548

DISCARDED

CONQUERING BLADDER AND PROSTATE PROBLEMS

The Authoritative Guide for Men and Women

Jerry G. Blaivas, M.D.

PERSEUS PUBLISHING

Cambridge, Massachusetts

COLLEGE OF THE SEQUOIAS
LIBRARY

Many of the disignations used by manufacturers and sellers to distinguish their products are claimed as trademarks. Where those designations appear in this book and Perseus Publishing was aware of a trademark claim, the designations have been printed in initial capital letters.

Copyright © 1998 by Jerry G. Blaivas

All rights reserved. No part of this publication may be reproduced, stored in a retrieval system, or transmitted, in any form or by any means, electronic, mechanical, photocopying, recording, or otherwise, without the prior written permission of the publisher. Printed in the United States of America.

CIP data is available at the Library of Congress.
ISBN 0-7382-0439-0

Perseus Publishing is a member of the Perseus Books Group.

Find us on the World Wide Web at http://www.perseuspublishing.com.

Perseus Publishing books are available at special discounts for bulk purchases in the U.S. by corporations, institutions, and other organizations. For more information, please contact the Special Markets Department at HarperCollins Publishers, 10 East 53rd Street, New York, NY 10022, or call 1-212-207-7528.

Set in 10-point Palatino by Perseus Publishing Services

First paperback printing

1 2 3 4 5 6 7 8 9 10–03 02 01

To my wife, Susan, friend and companion for life whose strength and character have seen us through the worst of times, and whose love and compassion have led us to the best of times.

And to my three daughters, my best friends, to whom she passed on all of the good genes: Heidi, Kimberly, and Lindsey.

Contents

Preface

This is a book written for people who have urinary bladder and prostate problems—people who urinate too often, who plan their daily activities around the availability of a bathroom; men with prostate problems; women with incontinence who wet their clothes without warning; and people with bladder pain.

The chances are that you have no idea how your bladder or prostate really works. You may question why you urinate so much, or why you lose control of your urine. You may experience pain in your bladder or your prostate (or what you think is your bladder or prostate), but not know what kind of a doctor to see, or what to expect, or what to ask.

The purpose of this book is to answer all these questions and many more.

HOW TO READ THIS BOOK

Not everyone will want, or even need, to read this book from start to finish. For example, if you are a woman you may not be interested in how the prostate works. If you have already been diagnosed with a bladder problem you may not be interested in diagnosis, but only in treatment options. That is why each chapter is designed to be a self-contained unit. You don't have to read the preceding chapters to understand the current one. However, this necessitates some repetition. Whenever you come across something that needs a little more explanation, you may be referred back to the original chapter where that topic was discussed in more detail. If you see a word that you don't recognize, look it up in the glossary.

If you have any interest in understanding how things work, what can go wrong, and what symptoms mean, I recommend that you read the first three chapters. It is my hope that this book will guide you in understanding and in making informed judgments on an array of disturbing and sometimes life-threatening conditions. Through such knowledge, you should expect effective treatment and an end to the symptoms that made you pick up this book in the first place.

One word of caution, though: When it comes to diagnosis and treatment, there are no hard-and-fast rules. The information you get from this book is intended to aid you in your consultation with your physician. But beware, do not be your own physician. Take heed of the old adage "the physician who treats himself has a fool for a patient."

Acknowledgments

When Isaac Newton was praised for his scientific accomplishments, he remarked, "If I have seen further, it is by standing on the shoulders of giants." I stand on a lot of shoulders and I'd like to thank you all.

First, my good friends and colleagues Edward J. McGuire, M.D., Shlomo Rax, M.D., and Alan J. Wein, M.D. You three have been the cornerstones of my intellectual, surgical, and personal development.

Professor of Urology at the University of Michigan, Ed McGuire has nearly single-handedly revolutionized the way doctors think about incontinence, neurogenic bladder, and other lower urinary tract disturbances. He has a unique ability to learn from his own experience, and I believe he has a kind of innate intuition about the way the urinary tract works. To Ed McGuire we owe our basic understanding of the causes of incontinence and how, as surgeons, we can fix them. On a personal level, I owe Ed McGuire a lot more. He taught me how to do a pubovaginal sling (and never lets me forget it).

Shlomo Rax, Professor of Urology at the University of California, Los Angeles, is a charismatic and inspiring surgeon, a great thinker, and an innovator. He is a good friend and a good person whose professionalism and surgical renown are blended with a deep sense of humanity. His name is synonymous with female urology.

Alan Wein is Professor and Chairman, Division of Urology, at the University of Pennsylvania School of Medicine. His intellect, professionalism, work ethic, leadership, and plain common sense humble the rest of us. And he is a good friend. His collaboration with Robert Levin, Ph.D., created one of the greatest urologic research efforts in history.

David M. Barrett, M.D., CEO of Lahey Clinic, is a gentleman, a surgeon, a leader, and a good friend.

Joseph N. Corriere Jr., M.D., is Professor of Surgery at the University of Texas Health Science Center at Houston and Director, American Urological Association, Office of Education. His work ethic, honesty, humanity, and devotion to education make up, in part, for his golf.

John O. L. DeLancey, M.D., Associate Professor and Chief of Gynecology at the University of Michigan Medical Center is a gynecologic physician and surgeon, an intellect and researcher par excellence. I thank him for his depiction of the anatomy and function of the female pelvic floor; I thank him for his humanity as well.

William Fair, M.D., former Florence and Theodore Baumritter/Enid Nacall Chairman of Urologic Surgery at Memorial Sloan Kettering Cancer Center, is a role model and an inspiration as a chairman, a scientist, a researcher, and a person.

Frank Hinman Jr., M.D., Clinical Professor of Urology, University of California, San Francisco is a surgeon, a scholar, a medical illustrator, an artist, and, most of all, a gentleman.

Neil Resnick, M.D., is Professor and Chief of Geriatric Medicine at the University of Pittsburgh School of Medicine. With a deep sense of humanity and scholarship, he teaches us about the unique problems of aging and how to care for older people.

Emil A. Tanagho, M.D., Professor of Urology, University of California, San Francisco epitomizes the surgical scholar and basic scientist.

Some others of you may not even know why you're included, but your contributions helped me to understand the complex ways in which the lower urinary tract works and how to fix it whem it malfunctions. Collectively you provided me with the knowledge to write a book like this—Alison Brading, M.A., Ph.D., B.S.C., Michael B. Chancellor, M.D., Bo Coolsaet, M.D., Ph.D., Ahmad Elbadawi, M.D., Tom Elkins, M.D., Derek Giffiths, Ph.D., Robert M. Levin, Ph.D., Alan Retik, M.D., Lauri Romanzi, M.D., Allain Rossier, M.D., Werner Shafer, Ph.D., Thomas A. Stamey, M.D., Patrick C. Walsh, M.D., Subbarao V. Yalla, M.D., and Leonard Zinman, M.D.

I had a lot of other help.

Heidi Blaivas, my friend, my confidante, and my daughter, did a yeoman's job, and was always there to pick up all of the pieces.

Leslie Oliver, RN. MBA, a consummate professional and friend for over 20 years, and Mike Verhaaren, LPN, were always there when I needed them.

Linda Regan, my editor, who gave me back each edited page faster than I wrote it, made sure than my written words conveyed their intended message.

My heartfelt thanks to you all.

CONQUERING BLADDER AND PROSTATE PROBLEMS

The Authoritative Guide for Men and Women

1

The Bladder and the Kidneys
All about Urine

Why is it that one perfectly healthy person feels the need to urinate every two to three hours during the day while another is quite comfortable going only once or twice all day? What actually causes the urge to urinate? Is it pressure? Is it bladder volume? Is it tension within the wall of the bladder? The answers to these seemingly simple questions have plagued scientists for decades and no simple answer is forthcoming. Nevertheless, some facts are clear. Neither pressure, nor volume, nor tension alone is responsible for the urge to urinate. Rather, it seems to be the combining of all three factors along with a multitude of environmental and psychological influences.

Consider, for example, your very own bladder. Let's say you've been hired as an expert at $100 per cup of coffee to participate in a coffee tasting marathon. The more you taste, the more money you make (and the more urine your kidneys produce). Of course, the more you drink, the more you urinate. Now remember, this is a coffee-tasting marathon. The organizers want your opinion as to the quality of the coffee. They want you to be relaxed and comfortable. Whenever you feel the urge to urinate you simply go into the bathroom and void. So you drink and you void, you drink and you void. You're in the bathroom about once an hour. All of a sudden, while talking with a fellow taste tester, you realize you have a particularly strong urge to urinate. While hurrying to the bathroom, you spy what looks like a horde of drug-crazed crack addicts bursting into the office in search of drug money. You catch their eye and they begin to chase you down the stairs and into the street. They chase you for two and a half hours, past stores and restaurants with bathrooms, and yet you never stop to void. In fact, you no longer even have the urge to urinate. Exhausted, you stop and they finally catch up to you. It turns out that these were not drug-crazed crack addicts at all, but lottery officials who inform you that you've just won the $12 million jackpot. Upon hearing this you pee in your pants.

Congratulations, but this is about urinating. Why did you urinate once per hour during the coffee-tasting marathon, then not urinate for over two and a half hours while being chased, then wet your pants when you won the lottery? It certainly wasn't due to bladder pressure or bladder volume or bladder wall tension. Somehow the same signals that were sent up to the brain from the bladder were altered in the three different situations. In the first scenario you were sitting comfortably, sipping coffee. Your kidneys made some urine and sent it to the bladder. As the bladder filled, its nerves were stimulated and sent chemical messages to the brain signaling that it was time to urinate. You leisurely arose, walked the ten steps to the bathroom and urinated. No problem.

In the second scenario you were preoccupied. Your kidneys had already produced a large volume of urine that was stored in your bladder when you finally heeded your brain's signal that it was time to void. You got up to go to the bathroom and suddenly found yourself running down the street. Your bladder was still filling up with urine and it was sending its chemical messengers up to the brain. But the messages were blocked by other messages from your eyes and ears that were telling your brain to "forget about the bathroom, it's time to get out of here."

In the third scenario you were so excited that you didn't even think about your bladder. You hit the jackpot and you were oblivious. In that instant, two and a half hours of stored up chemical messages, screaming "it's time to go, it's time to go," hit your brain all at once and you urinated all over the floor.

URINE

What is urine? What is its purpose? How much urine does your body make? Can you make too much or too little urine? Can you do anything to regulate the amount of urine that is produced? Let us look at the answers to these and some other questions.

WHAT IS URINE?

Urine is the liquid waste product of the body. It is produced by the kidneys, which filter dissolved waste from the bloodstream and store it in the bladder. The kidneys are remarkable organs that carefully regulate your body chemistry and the amount of fluid in your body. The kidneys maintain a balance between the amount of fluid you ingest and the amount of fluid lost from your skin (sweat), intestines (diarrhea), and lungs (the breath you exhale may contain large amounts of fluid in the form of vapor). Unless there are excessive losses of fluids due to sweating or diseases that cause diarrhea, the rate of urine production by the kidneys depends mostly on how much you eat and drink.

HOW MUCH URINE DOES THE BODY MAKE?

It's very simple; the more you eat and drink, the more urine the kidneys produce and the more time you spend in the bathroom. Conversely, the less you drink and eat, the less urine you make. Normally, the kidneys produce urine at a rate of about 30–100 ml per hour (1–3 oz. per hour), depending mostly on the type and amount of fluid you ingest. For example, if you drink an excessive amount of coffee, there is a dual effect on urine production. The amount of coffee that you drink contributes to your total intake of fluid and thus the amount of water that enters your system. In addition, coffee contains caffeine, which is a diuretic—a substance that increases the rate of urine production. So if you drink coffee, your kidneys will produce more urine than they would if you drank an equal amount of fluid not containing caffeine. Coffee drinking is not harmful, but it does cause you to urinate more often.

Your body does not manufacture fluid; all the fluid comes from conversion of what you eat and drink. Thus, except for the symptoms of certain disease states that impair the kidneys' ability to regulate urine output, it is impossible to produce more urine than the sum of the fluid that you ingest by drinking and eating. If you do urinate more fluid than you take in, you become dehydrated, like a raisin (a dehydrated grape) or a prune (a dehydrated plum). If dehydration persists for more than a few weeks your body chemistry becomes deranged and, without proper treatment, you shrivel up (like a grape) and die. You simply can't continually urinate more than the sum of all the fluid you ingest without becoming very ill. Under ordinary circumstances, this never happens, but there are rare conditions, such as diabetes insipidus or starvation, that result in such severe dehydration, leading to death.

HOW MUCH SHOULD YOU DRINK?

Unless you have severe kidney damage, the best guide to how much to drink is your own thirst. Thirst is the basic means by which the body regulates its internal fluid requirements. The sensation of thirst occurs when there is not enough water in your body or when there is relatively too much salt.

Actually, it's a bit more complicated than this. Believe it or not, your body is mostly composed of water. If you're fat, you're about 50% water; if you're skinny, you're about 70% water. The water is unevenly distributed throughout your body, divided amongst two major compartments—the intracellular and extracellular spaces. The whole body is made up of millions of individual microscopic cells. Each cell is composed of at least 50% water. The intracellular space is the sum of all of the spaces within all of the cells of the body. The extracellular space is the sum of all the spaces between cells. There are lots of things dissolved in the water in your body, but mostly electrolytes and proteins. Electrolytes are molecules like sodium, chloride, and potassium (table salt is sodium chloride). The intracellular and extracellular spaces are separated by cell membranes that are semipermeable, which means that, although water can move freely across the membrane, some substances cannot and are stuck in one compartment or the other. Semipermeable membranes actually have tiny holes in them like a piece of Swiss cheese. Some particles, like sodium and chloride, can easily fit through the holes; others, like large proteins, cannot.

So both the intracellular and extracellular spaces are filled with water and dissolved proteins and electrolytes. The two spaces are separated by semipermeable membranes. Water can move freely between the spaces, but some of the dissolved substances cannot. Imagine a cardboard box, divided in half by a large piece of Swiss cheese. On one side are large moths; on the other are mosquitos. The moths are like the proteins in your body; they cannot fit through the holes and must stay on one side. The mosquitos are like electrolytes; they can easily fit through the holes and eventually fly through and inhabit both sides of the box. So the moths (proteins) stay on one side and the mosquitos (electrolytes) fly freely on both sides. The extracellular space has both proteins (moths) and electrolytes (mosquitos), and the intracellular space contains mostly electrolytes. Water moves freely through the cell wall (the semipermeable membrane).

If you don't drink enough, or if you lose too much water through sweating or diarrhea, you become dehydrated (your body has insufficient water) and this causes you to be thirsty. Thirst is normally caused by an increase in extracellular osmotic pressure (that means there isn't enough water in the extracellular space). When this happens, you need to drink until enough water gets into the extracellular space and you're back in balance.

The average person drinks about 1.2 liters (a little more than a quart) of fluid each day and takes in another liter in his or her food. However, if there are abnormal losses of fluid from sweating, diarrhea, vomiting, blood loss, etc., you may need to drink a lot more to stay in balance. The old adage that you must drink at least eight glasses of fluid per day is nothing more than an old wives' tale. Thirst is the best guide to how much you should drink. In fact, if you do drink eight glasses of fluid per day, you'll probably spend a lot of time in the bathroom. If your bladder normally holds about a glass, you'll be urinating eight times a day; if it holds only half a glass, you'll be urinating sixteen times per day.

Of course, there are many reasons other than thirst why you might drink a lot of fluid—your overall health requires that you pay attention to more than just your kidneys. You might need to drink a lot of fluids for certain kinds of diets, to help with digestion, to hydrate your skin, or for a variety of other kinds of conditions. For example, people who are prone to kidney stones are encouraged to drink large amounts of fluids every day. It's recommended that they drink a glass of water before they go to bed at night and then another when they are awakened in the middle of the night to urinate. That is the best way to prevent kidney stones. Having kidney stones is very painful; passing them is said to be more painful than childbirth, so people are willing to put up with a lot to prevent them. But drinking that much fluid has its price—you urinate very frequently.

HOW OFTEN SHOULD I URINATE?

Although you may get the urge to urinate a number of times throughout the day, the urge is normally neither painful nor uncomfortable and can usually be comfortably postponed for at least a half hour or more. In fact, most people can postpone the need to void for two or three or more hours once they perceive the urge. The bladder can normally hold at least 200–600 ml (7–20 oz.) before the urge to urinate becomes uncomfortable. On average, people urinate approximately every three to five hours during the day (five to seven times) and sleep through the night without voiding, although many normal people get up once or twice at night to urinate. However, the actual amount and frequency of urination is very much dependent on (1) how much urine your kidneys produce and (2) how comfortable it is for your bladder to hold or store the urine.

CONCLUSION

Urine is the liquid waste product of the body produced by the kidneys, which serve as a filter for all of the fluid and dissolved substances in the blood. The kidneys filter the blood and excrete the extra water and dissolved substances (protein and electrolytes) as urine. Urine is made in the kidneys and stored in the bladder. When the bladder becomes full, you urinate.

The best guide as to how much fluid to drink is your own thirst. If you do not drink enough (or you lose an excessive amount of fluid through sweating or diarrhea), your kidneys cut down on urine production to conserve water and you get thirsty and drink. If you drink more than you need, the kidneys make more urine to keep you in balance.

How often you urinate depends on two factors—how much urine your kidneys make and how much urine your bladder can hold. The more you drink, the more urine your kidneys make, and the more often you urinate; the less your bladder can hold, the more often you urinate.

2

Anatomy of the Urinary System
and How It Works

The urinary system consists of the two kidneys, the ureters, the bladder, and the urethra (Figures 1–3). The two kidneys lie in the back, just in front of the lower rib cage on either side of the spinal cord. Urine made by the kidneys is transported to the bladder by the two ureters, where it is stored until it is urinated. Each *ureter* is a thin, hollow, muscular tube that connects the kidney to the bladder. The *bladder*, a hollow muscular organ whose purpose is to store urine, is connected to the tip of the penis in men and to the upper vagina in women by another thin muscular tube called the *urethra*. In the wall of the urethra is a very efficient group of muscles collectively known as the *urethral sphincter*. The sphincter keeps the urethra tightly closed to prevent the involuntary loss of urine (incontinence). The act of urination is accomplished when the bladder contracts and the sphincter relaxes, forcing urine out the urethra.

In the male, another organ, the *prostate*, surrounds and lies in the wall of the urethra just at its connection with the bladder. Imagine that you took a straw and passed it through the center of an apple. The straw is like the urethra; the apple is like the prostate. The prostate does not appear to have a very important role and men can live a normal life without a prostate. Some people think it's just there to keep urologists busy. About the only thing we know for sure is that it does make prostatic fluid which mixes with sperm during the sexual act, and it does provide some protection against infection. In the female, the urethra is quite short, only about an inch long. It opens into the upper part of the vagina, just below the clitoris and underneath the pubic bone (Figure 4). The bladder and urethra

7

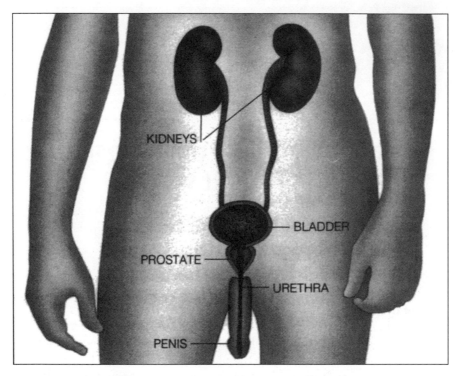

Figure 1. Anatomy of the urinary system in the male—front view. Courtesy of the American Foundation of Urologic Disease.

are supported by a hammocklike structure known as the pelvic floor muscles. These muscles are attached to the bones of the pelvis and suspend the bladder, urethra, vagina, and rectum from the bony side walls of the pelvis (Figure 5).

To better visualize how this works, put your hands together in your lap, palms up and fingers interlocking. Put your two thumbs together to form an upside-down V. Your palms and fingers represent the pelvic floor muscles. The bladder rests on these muscles and the urethra goes through the arch of the upside-down V.

HOW THE BLADDER WORKS

The bladder serves as a reservoir for urine and provides a means for its elimination. At first glance, it seems like a rather simple setup. The

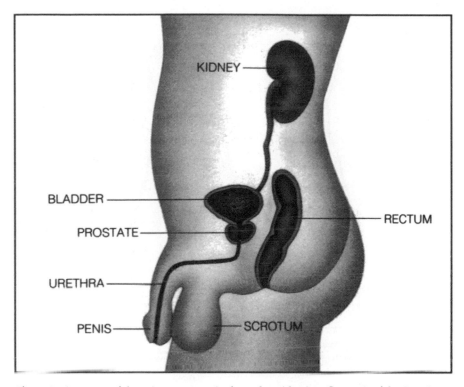

Figure 2. Anatomy of the urinary system in the male—side view. Courtesy of the American Foundation of Urologic Disease.

bladder might be considered to be like a balloon and the urethra like the narrow end where air is blown in. The knot tied in the stem of the balloon, which prevents air from escaping, is similar to the sphincter muscle that prevents urine from escaping. When the balloon is full, no air escapes as long as the knot is securely tied. To empty the balloon, all one need do is undo the knot and the air rushes out. If the knot (sphincter) is tied too loosely or not at all, air can leak out when you don't want it to. In a similar way, if the sphincter muscles are weak, urine may leak from the bladder. This is called *incontinence*. If the sphincter is obstructed, or if there is a narrowing of the urethra, the result is a blockage in the flow of urine. This causes the urinary stream to be weak, and if the blockage is very severe, you might not be able to urinate at all.

Actually, the bladder isn't exactly like a balloon, and the sphincter isn't exactly like a knot; they are more complicated than that. If you want to find out more, read on. The bladder is a hollow, muscular sac composed

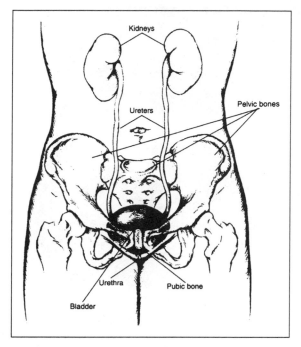

Figure 3. Anatomy of the urinary system in the female—front view. Courtesy of the American Urologic Association.

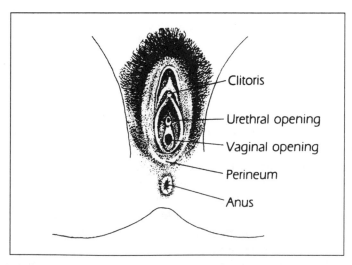

Figure 4. Anatomy of the vagina and urethral meatus (opening). From W. Smith, *Overcoming Cystitis: A Practical Self-Help Guide for Women,* Bantam Books, New York, 1987, with permission.

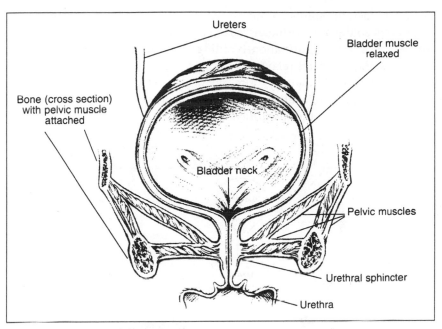

Figure 5. Anatomy of the female pelvis and pelvic muscles. Courtesy of the American Urological Association.

of intertwining smooth muscle fibers, an extracellular matrix between the muscle cells, and an inner lining called the mucosa. The *mucosa* is similar to the lining of the inside of your mouth, but it is composed of a different kind of cell called a transitional cell; hence, the bladder is said to be lined by mucosa composed of transitional cell epithelium. The mucosa serves as a natural barrier to infection. The smooth muscle of the bladder is called the *detrusor*. It is called an involuntary muscle because we ordinarily cannot control its minute-to-minute activity. It's the same kind of muscle that is in the intestines. The extracellular matrix is the structural architecture around which the bladder is formed.

As the bladder fills with urine, the pressure on its walls remains very low because of a unique property of its wall known as *accommodation*, which refers to the ability of the bladder gradually to accept larger and larger amounts of urine without increasing its pressure. If the bladder behaved like a balloon, the inside pressure would continue to build up and eventually become so great that the bladder would either burst or there would be leakage of urine through the urethra. As the bladder continues to fill with urine, the sphincter muscle around the urethra remains tightly

closed. In fact, the sphincter muscle actually increases its contraction during filling, so the more urine there is in the bladder, the tighter the sphincter becomes. During urination (voiding) the bladder muscle (detrusor)
contracts, the sphincter relaxes and opens, and urine is expelled through
the urethra and (hopefully) into the toilet. This orderly sequence of
events—sphincter relaxation, detrusor contraction, and the onset of urinary flow—is called the *micturition reflex* (Figure 6).

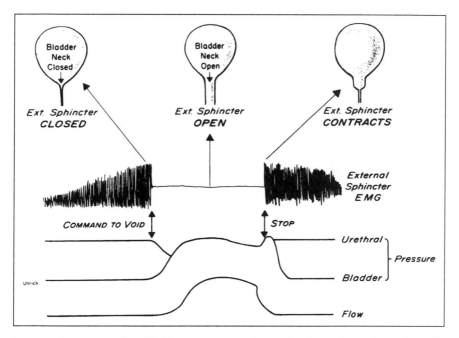

Figure 6. Physiology of the bladder and the micturition reflex. Normally, as the bladder fills
with urine from the kidneys, the pressure in the bladder remains low and fairly constant.
The pressure in the urethra remains greater than the pressure in the bladder, and the bladder
neck and external sphincter urethral remain closed so that leakage of urine does not occur.
The electrical activity of the sphincter muscles, known as the electromyographic (EMG) activity, gradually increases as the bladder fills. Urination begins with a sudden and complete
relaxation of the external sphincter, evident as a cessation of EMG activity and a fall in the
pressure in the urethra (marked on this tracing as Command to Void). The urethra opens
widely as the sphincter relaxes. Almost immediately, the bladder begins to contract, seen as a
rise in bladder pressure, and urine begins to flow, evident on the urine flow tracing. Urination ceases with contraction of the muscles of the external urethral sphincter (marked at the
arrow indicating Stop). The contracting sphincter cuts off the urinary stream and this causes
a momentary rise in urethral and bladder pressure. Within seconds, the bladder stops contracting. From J. G. Blaivas, "Pathophysiology of Lower Urinary Tract Dysfunction," *Urologic
Clinics of North America*, 12:215, 1985, with permission.

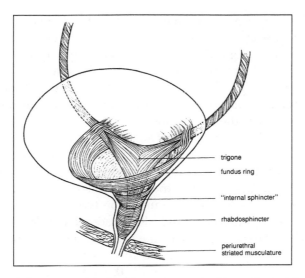

trigone

fundus ring

"internal sphincter"

rhabdosphincter

periurethral
striated musculature

Figure 7. Detailed anatomy of the bladder, ureters, and sphincter. See text for discussion.

Although the urethra functions as a sphincter, the sphincter cannot be seen with the naked eye. Nor is it apparent under the careful scrutiny of the microscope or even in the gross anatomy laboratory. There is no valve, like there is in the heart. Rather, the function of the urethra as a sphincter results from an integrated interaction between smooth (involuntary) and striated (voluntary) muscle inside and around the urethral wall and other components of the soft tissue including collagen and elastin, and a mucosal seal.

The junction between the urethra and the bladder is called the *bladder neck*. Its wall is composed mostly of smooth muscle that is arranged in both a circular and longitudinal pattern around the urethra (Figure 7). The smooth muscle of the urethra is called the *internal sphincter*. Wrapped around the smooth muscle, the striated muscle in the wall of the urethra is called the *rhabdosphincter* and the striated muscle surrounding the urethra is called the *periurethral striated muscle*. Together they form the *external urethral sphincter*.

Coming from the kidneys, the ureters pierce the bladder wall at an oblique angle and continue in the wall for about 2 cm (about an inch). Then they pierce the mucosa and form the ureteral orifices (the entrances of the ureters into the bladder). The muscles of the ureters are arranged in spiral fashion until they reach the bladder. At the outside of the bladder, the muscles assume a longitudinal configuration. Urine made in the kidneys is transported down the ureters and enters the bladder through the ureteral orifices. The muscle in the wall of the ureter does not stop at the ureteral orifice. Rather, it continues into the wall of the bladder, fans out and meets the ureteral muscle from the other ureter and continues down the urethra as the longitudinal smooth muscle layer of the urethra. The part of the urethra that fans out forms a triangular-shaped plate of smooth muscle called the *trigone* (Bell's muscle). Another layer of muscle, in the wall of the bladder (the *fundus ring*), surrounds the trigone and is part of the smooth muscle of the bladder neck.

It is actually the arrangement of all of these structures that constitutes the external urethral sphincter. It works like this: During the storage phase, as the bladder is filling with urine from the kidneys, the smooth muscles of the bladder neck and striated muscles of the external sphincter remain closed (Figure 8A). During urination (voiding) the smooth muscles of the ureter and trigone, and the longitudinal muscles of the urethra, contract. This shortens and widens the urethra, and, in conjunction with relaxation of the external sphincter, the urethra opens widely (Figure 8B). As the trigonal muscle contracts, it pulls the ureteral orifices downward and inward. This stretching of the ureters narrows them and as the bladder contracts, its walls are compressed, preventing backup of urine to the ureters and kidneys. In some disease states this valvelike mechanism is faulty and there is backup of urine into the ureters and kidneys, known as *vesicoureteral reflux*.

In the bladder and urethra, the extracellular matrix, composed mostly of collagen, gives structural support to the tissues (like the framework of a house). Elastin in the extracellular matrix helps bind the tissues together and keeps the urethra closed during the storage phase. The mucosal seal is similar to caulking used to prevent water leaks around window panes.

Control of the bladder and sphincter is regulated by at least three different parts of the nervous system: (1) the pons (pontine micturition center), which is in the lower part of the brain just above the spinal cord; (2) the thoracolumbar (middle) portion of the spinal cord; and (3) the sacral (sacral micturition center) portion of the spinal cord, located in its lower portion (Figure 9).

The nervous system has two main divisions—the autonomic and somatic nervous systems. The autonomic system controls involuntary bodily functions such as breathing, the heartbeat, and the functions of the bladder. The nerve supply to all smooth muscle comes from the autonomic nervous system. The autonomic nervous system is further subdivided into the parasympathetic and sympathetic nervous systems. The somatic nervous system regulates voluntary functions such as the movement of your arms and legs and the voluntary muscles of the urethra. The nerve supply to all voluntary (striated) muscles comes from the somatic nervous system.

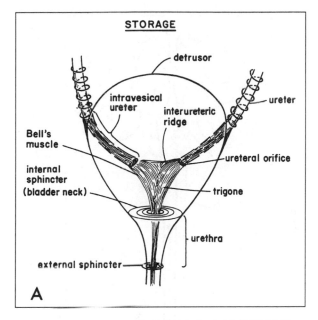

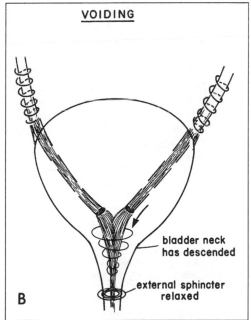

Figure 8. Functional anatomy of the bladder, sphincter, and ureters;   A, storage phase;   B, voiding. See text for explanation. From J. G. Blaivas and J. D. Ferrone, "Urologic Complications in the Critically Ill Orthopedic Patient," *Orthopedic Clinics of North America,* 9:825, 1978, with permission.

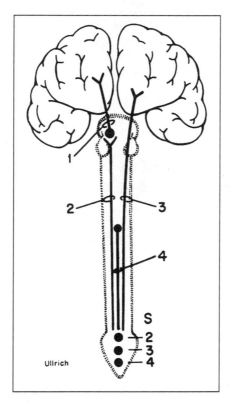

Figure 9. Neurologic control of the bladder and sphincter. The micturition reflex is coordinated by the pontine micturition center (PMC), located in the pons, a part of the brain just above the spinal cord. The PMC is marked by a black circle at pathway 1. The pontine micturition center sends and receives messages from the sacral micturition center (SMC), which is located in the sacral portion of the spinal cord in sacral segments (S2–4). The connection between the PMC and SMC is pathway 2 in this diagram. When neurologic disease interrupts this pathway, the micturition reflex becomes uncoordinated, a condition known as detrusor sphincter dyssynergia. Voluntary control of micturition is accomplished by connections between many different parts of the brain and the PMC (pathway 1). When these pathways are damaged, voluntary control of micturition is lost and the person develops urinary incontinence. The SMC and the thoracolumbar center contain the nerves that make the bladder and sphincter contract and relax under the control of the PMC (pathway 4). Another set of connections, between a part of the brain called the frontal cortex and the SMC (pathway 3), is necessary for a person to contract his or her sphincter to stop the urinary stream or to prevent urination. From J. G. Blaivas, "Pathophysiology of Lower Urinary Tract Dysfunction," *Urologic Clinics of North America,* 12:215, 1985, with permission.

Muscles and nerves communicate with one another via chemical messengers called neurotransmitters. Neurotransmitters are released from the ends of nerves (terminals) and then pass through a connection between either another nerve or a muscle where, among other things, they may instruct the muscle to contract or relax. There are many different types of neurotransmitters. The most ubiquitous one is called *acetylcholine*. It is used by both the autonomic and somatic nervous systems. *Norepinephrine* is the next most common neurotransmitter, but it is used only by the autonomic nervous system. Acetylcholine is the neurotransmitter that makes the bladder contract. Acetylcholine and medications that mimic its effects are called *cholinergic agonists*. Medications that block the action of acetylcholine are called *anticholinergics*. Anticholinergics are often prescribed for patients who have urinary incontinence because of involuntary contractions of the bladder. Norepinephrine is the neurotransmitter that keeps the urethra closed. If the actions of norepinephrine are overactive, it can cause prostatic or bladder neck obstruction. Norepinephrine and medications that mimic its actions are called *alpha-adrenergic agonists*. Medications that block the effects of norepinephrine are called *alpha-adrenergic antagonists*, or *alpha blockers*. Alpha blockers are often used to treat prostatic obstruction.

Infants have no control over urination—the *micturition reflex* (relaxation of the sphincter, contraction of the bladder, opening of the urethra, and the onset of urination) is activated when the bladder gets full and the baby urinates. With the passage of time, we all learn to control our bladders, with a little help from our parents. By the end of the toddler years, most children have normal daytime control, and by age ten nearly all have nighttime control as well. People who are born with neurologic conditions like spina bifida may never learn to control their bladders, and normal people who develop neurologic conditions such as multiple sclerosis and stroke may lose bladder control. Fortunately, when this happens there is effective treatment for the great majority of people.

CONCLUSION

The urinary system consists of the kidneys, ureters, bladder, and urethra. In the wall of the urethra are specialized muscles that constitute the sphincter. Urination is under the control of the nervous system and when neurologic diseases occur, control of urination may be lost.

3

Bladder Symptoms

Lisa, a 41-year-old secretary, while working at her desk, felt a sudden urge to urinate. She rushed to bathroom and by the time she got there, she had an intense pain in her lower abdomen. When she tried to void, only a few drops came out. She went back to her desk and five minutes later, the same thing happened. This time the urine was red; it looked like blood. She went to her doctor, who diagnosed a bladder infection and prescribed antibiotics. She felt better within eight hours.

Six years ago, Lisa's mother had exactly the same symptoms. She went to the same doctor and he told her she had a urinary tract infection. She was treated with antibiotics and the symptoms got better. One month later, the symptoms recurred and she was diagnosed with bladder cancer. She underwent surgery to remove the tumor and now she's fine.

John is a 46-year-old barber. He began to urinate very frequently and sometimes felt a stinging pain at the tip of his penis. It turned out that he had a kidney stone.

One of John's customers, Bill, a 61-year-old doctor himself, had almost identical symptoms to John. He tried treating himself with antibiotics with no results. He saw a urologist, who discovered that, in Bill's case, urine was backing up because of an enlarged prostate. Bill required an operation so that he could urinate normally again. Along the way, he learned the old adage, "a doctor who treats himself has a fool for a patient."

Bill had a patient, Sam, a 63-year-old retired fireman, who had the same symptoms, so Bill sent him to the same urologist, because he thought that Sam too had an enlarged prostate. However, Sam had kidney cancer.

By now it should seem obvious that the bladder has a rather limited means of expressing its own pathology. No matter what is wrong, there are only five sets of symptoms that encompass all of the known conditions that affect the bladder. These symptoms are (1) urinary frequency, urgency, and nocturia (urinating at night); (2) loss of urinary control (incontinence); (3) pain; (4) difficulty urinating or the inability to urinate at all (urinary retention); and (5) blood in the urine.

A disabling, unrelenting pain can be caused by a simple bladder infection; a seemingly trivial complaint, like frequency of urination, can be caused by a serious condition like bladder or prostate cancer. How do you know what's wrong? How do you even known when to see a doctor? These questions will be answered in the next chapter, but first you need to know what the symptoms are and what they can mean.

URINARY FREQUENCY, URGENCY, AND NOCTURIA

How often should you urinate? As we mentioned earlier, it all depends on how much you drink. The more you drink, the more urine your kidneys produce and the more you have to urinate. The frequency of urination and the associated sensations are also dependent on a complex interaction between the signals that the bladder sends out and the signals that the brain receives from other environmental and psychosocial sources. There is no simple definition of urinary frequency because some people are perfectly comfortable going to the bathroom every hour for the sake of convenience, whereas others find it very distressing to have to interrupt what they are doing more than three or four times per day to urinate. Thus, in part, it is not how often you urinate, but why and how you react to the frequency of urination that determines whether or not it is a "symptom."

There are no strict values for normal and abnormal, but, on average, most people ingest approximately 1500–2000 ml of fluid per day ($1^1/_2$–2 qt.) and void a total of about 1000–2500 ml (1–$2^1/_2$ qt.) of urine per 24 hours. The volume of each urination is also variable. Some people void only 100–200 ml at a time; others void as much as 1000 ml or more at a time. Thus, depending on the amount of urine that your bladder can comfortably hold before you feel the need to urinate, it is possible to urinate as little as two to three times per day or as much as once an hour, yet still pass the same total amount of urine. Most normal people, though, urinate about once very three to five hours during the day and most are not awakened more than once a night by the urge to urinate once they go to sleep.

Nocturia literally means "urinating at night." Sometimes it is a symptom; sometimes it is not. If you're awakened every hour once you go to sleep because of the urge to urinate, that's a symptom. If you're worried about something and you can't sleep, and you drink tea or milk to help you sleep and you get up every hour to urinate, that's a symptom of worry, but it's not a bladder problem. If you are a night watchman (or a night watch-woman) and you're up all night, it's normal to urinate at night and it's not a symptom, but if you're up all day urinating, when you're supposed to be sleeping, that's a symptom. As you might have guessed, the most common reason why people get up at night to urinate is that their kidneys make a lot of urine at night, so the bladder responds the way it is supposed to, by waking them up and telling them to urinate.

The single most common cause of urinary frequency is probably a learned behavior, or a bad habit. Other common causes include excessive oral intake of fluid, urinary tract infection, a hypersensitive bladder, prostate problems, and bladder cancer. A more complete list of the causes of urinary frequency, urgency, and nocturia is seen in Table 1.

Urinary urgency is defined as the feeling that urination is imminent and that if you don't get to the bathroom in time you will either lose control and wet yourself or there will be considerable pain or discomfort. Occasional urinary urgency is normal. For example, if you delay urination too long after the initial urge is felt, a feeling of growing urgency is normal. Thus, urinary frequency and urgency may be caused by a variety of different pathological conditions or may simply be the result of drinking too much fluid and delaying urination.

Table 1. Causes of Urinary Frequency, Urgency, and Nocturia

1. Excessive amount of urine output
   A. Excessive fluid intake (you drink or eat too much)
      1. Learned behavior or bad habit
      2. Diabetes mellitus
      3. Psychological reasons
   B. Abnormal production of urine by the kidneys
      1. Diabetes insipidus (the kidneys make too much urine)
         a. Neurogenic causes (brain tumor, brain injury)
         b. Kidney disease
2. Reduced bladder capacity
   A. Urinary tract infection
   B. Attempts to prevent incontinence
   C. Interstitial cystitis and sensory urgency
   D. Enlarged prostate (in men)
   E. Bladder cancer
   F. Prostate cancer (in men)
   G. Neurogenic bladder (multiple sclerosis, stroke, Parkinson's disease, etc.)

URINARY INCONTINENCE

Urinary incontinence means the loss of urinary control. In the most severe cases, you may simply urinate without knowing it at all and find your clothes suddenly saturated. Or you may get a sudden urge to urinate when you put your key in the front door and leak on the way to the bathroom because you can't get there in time. You may lose a few drops of urine when you run and jump or you may lose a gush of urine when you cough or sneeze.

Incontinence is very embarrassing. It can make you feel unclean or it can make you smell of urine. It can be a severe problem that can make you fearful of even leaving your house. But it's treatable and curable. If you wet yourself now, you don't have to wet yourself in the future if you get proper treatment.

There are many causes of incontinence. They're discussed in much more detail in Chapters 5 and 8, but before you go to those chapters, you might want to read this simple explanation. If you wet yourself there are only three possible causes—either the bladder contracts when it is not supposed to, or the sphincter relaxes when it's not supposed to, or there's a hole in your bladder.

There could be a hole in my bladder? How could I get a hole in my bladder?

I'm not suggesting that you have a hole in your bladder. You likely don't have a hole in your bladder, because if you did, you wouldn't be reading about this, you'd already know there was a hole in your bladder. A hole in the bladder is called a *fistula*. The only way you can get a hole in the bladder is just after surgery (of the bladder or uterus) or after childbirth or after radiation to the lower abdomen for cancer. Even if you do have a fistula, it can always be repaired.

PAIN

Pain is impossible to define; it can only be described. Pain from the bladder and urethra is variously described as pressure, burning, aching, stinging, searing . . . the list is endless. Some pains are characteristic of a bladder or urethral problem; others are too vague to be used as symptoms.

The most common pain is that which is due to a urinary tract infection. It usually begins with a severe urgency, a need to rush to the bathroom. When you get there, as you start to urinate, you feel a burning sensation. The burning is usually felt in the urethra, but most people don't know exactly where their urethra is. In women, the urethra opens into the upper part of the vagina, about an inch below the clitoris (see Chapter 2, Figure 4). In men the urethral opening is at the tip of the penis. The burning or stinging usually lasts a few seconds after urination is complete, but then very often it begins again with an urgent need to urinate, often within a few minutes. Even though all of the above are the classic symptoms of *cystitis* (bacterial infection of the bladder), not all patients with these symptoms actually have a bacterial infection. In fact, about half the time, there is no identifiable infection as such and many physicians believe that these symptoms are due to viral infections that cannot be detected so easily. In rare cases, these same symptoms may be due to more serious conditions, such as bladder cancer and bladder stones in women and prostate conditions in men, which I will discuss later.

Many patients complain of bloating or aching in the lower abdomen that is not clearly related to urination. It is very difficult to diagnose the cause of this kind of discomfort with precision. There are lots of other organs and tissues near the bladder that can cause such symptoms—the rectum and lower end of the intestines, the uterus and ovaries, the muscles and other supporting tissues, and the nerves that innervate them. Even though the symptoms may have nothing to do with the bladder or with urination, many patients think they do, so they begin to urinate more frequently in a conscious attempt to diminish the pain. This can be very confusing to the doctor, because he or she thinks the pain is from the bladder, as does the patient. In fact, the pain may be coming from any or all those other organs, often requiring a fairly sophisticated evaluation to determine the cause and the treatment. No matter what, though, in the vast majority of patients the exact cause of the symptoms can be determined and effective treatment instituted.

There is one other kind of pain that is quite characteristic of a bladder problem. It's a pain that gets worse and worse if you don't urinate. Typically, the pain is described as a pressure or aching or sometimes a burning, which gets worse and worse the more you delay urination and immediately subsides as soon as you urinate, only to begin again and gradually get worse and worse until you urinate again. This is truly a bladder or urethral pain that has many causes, the most common of which is simply cystitis. Sometimes, after an episode of cystitis, the bladder "remembers" how painful it was and it continues to give the signal to urinate even after the infection is cured. Because of this, you urinate more frequently even though there is no obvious reason why. The more frequently you urinate, the more uncomfortable it becomes if you don't urinate, and a vicious cycle is started wherein frequent urination leads to even more frequent urina-

Table 2. Common Reasons for Pain in
the Region of the Bladder

Caused by bladder
   Urinary tract infection
   Bladder infection
   Prostate infection
   Urethral infection
   Urethral diverticulum
   Bladder or prostate cancer
   Bladder or kidney stones
   Urinary retention
   Interstitial cystitis
   Learned voiding dysfunction
Caused gynecologically
   Prolapse (dropped bladder)
   Endometriosis
   Vulvar vestibulitis
   Uterine fibroids
   Uterine and cervical cancer
   Ovarian cysts or cancer
Caused by rectum and intestine
   Hemorrhoids
   Anal fissure or fistula
   Irritable bowels syndrome
   Cancer of the colon
   Crohn's disease
Caused by muscle and nerve problems
   Herniated discs
   Neuropathies
   Muscle spasms

---

tion. Unless you train your bladder to hold more, you could actually end up being held hostage by your bladder, spending your life either in the bathroom or looking for a bathroom because of the discomfort felt if urination is postponed. Fortunately, in most cases there is very effective treatment for this problem. Table 2 lists the causes of pain in the bladder area.

DIFFICULTY URINATING AND URINARY RETENTION

Normally, urination is an effortless, almost unconscious act. You perceive the urge to urinate and, at a socially convenient time, go to the bathroom. Normal urination is accomplished almost immediately without pushing or straining, without hesitation, and in most instances, without any conscious effort at all. There are a number of symptoms that can occur during the act of *micturition* (urination)—*hesitancy* (a delay in starting), weak or dribbling urinary stream, *intermittency* (a starting–stopping urinary flow), a feeling of incomplete bladder emptying, a dribbling or dripping of urine after you think you are done, and, the most dramatic and frightening symptom, the inability to urinate at all. These symptoms are all nonspecific, which means that each symptom may be caused by a number of conditions. It is impossible to know what is wrong with you just by knowing what your symptoms are without doing more tests. For example, urinating with a weak or dribbling stream could be due to a blockage in the urethra, a weak bladder, or your own inability to relax. Each of these things can, in turn, be caused by many other conditions that require further evaluation to diagnose.

Hesitancy is defined as a delay in the time from the onset of the attempt to urinate until urine actually starts to flow. If you get the urge to urinate, go to the bathroom, and then have to wait before you are able to pass urine, you have hesitancy. Occasional hesitancy is normal; in fact, many people have hesitancy if they try to urinate before their bladder is full. Most people, when they notice that it is taking too long to start urination, begin to push or strain in an attempt to help it along. Others are able to void more easily when they hear the sound of running water (they simply turn on the faucet). Once the flow of urine starts there should be a rapid increase in the rate of flow, manifested by a forceful urinary stream, that continues until the bladder is completely empty. A weak or dribbling urinary stream is abnormal and may be due to (1) a blockage in the urethra (usually caused by an enlarged prostate, (2) a weak bladder contraction or no contraction at all, (3) a small volume of voided urine, or (4) a learned behavior wherein you are unable to relax the sphincter sufficiently to urinate normally.

If the urine fails to come out in a smooth, continuous flow, but rather comes out in spurts, the stream is said to be intermittent and the symptom is called intermittency. Intermittency may be due to alternately straining and relaxing during attempts to pass urine or voluntary or involuntary contractions of the sphincter muscle during urination. This condition may be either a learned behavior or a neurologic condition called *detrusor–sphincter dyssynergia* (dee-troo-sor/sfinkter/diss-sin-urg-ia) that is usually a result of either multiple sclerosis or spinal cord injury.

A feeling of incomplete bladder emptying may be due to just that; namely, there is residual urine left in the bladder after urination. However, not uncommonly, patients complain of incomplete bladder emptying, yet when tested they are found to have no residual urine at all. The cause of this symptom is simply not known at this time.

Postvoid dribbling is a common condition that is often seen in patients with urethral obstruction, particularly in men with prostatic obstruction. The reason for the postvoid dribbling is not clear. However, many normal women have postvoid dribbling for a very simple reason. During urination, a small amount of the urine gets trapped in the vagina. After they complete urination, when standing or straining, the urine is forced out of the vagina and accounts for the postvoid dribbling. There is a similar condition in men, wherein a few drops of urine remain in the widest portion of the urethra after urination. When they stand or strain there is leakage of those few drops. In men it is possible for them to "milk out" the last few drops; women may accomplish the same thing by wiping inside the vagina.

A most dramatic and frightening symptom is the sudden inability to urinate. Many patients with this condition have had years of warning—progressive difficulty urinating that culminates in acute urinary retention—but some patients have no warning at all. The symptoms of acute urinary retention are obvious. The patient is unable to urinate despite a severe and painful urge. In some people an urge is not felt; rather, they feel only severe pain in the lower abdomen. Not uncommonly there is also a burning sensation at the tip of the penis in men and a feeling that they "are going to burst." In most patients examination of the abdomen discloses a painful, distended bladder. The only treatment is to pass a small tube, or *catheter*, through the urethra into the bladder. This procedure allows urination and provides immediate relief of the pain, but only temporarily solves the problem. (The physician or nurse who actually passes the catheter has, more often than not, made a friend for life.) Once the emergency has passed, it will be necessary to determine the cause of the urinary retention and institute treatment so that it doesn't recur. Until an effective treatment is found it will be necessary to either leave the catheter in place or begin a program of *self intermittent catheterization* (SIC). Intermittent catheterization is a technique of managing your bladder when you can't urinate properly and don't empty sufficiently. Instead of urinating, you pass a catheter through the urethra to empty the urine. Almost all people who need it learn to do this usually pain-free procedure themselves and don't require any help. Each time, before you catheterize yourself, you try to urinate first. If you're able to urinate, eventually you'll be able to discontinue the SIC, but this should not be done until you've arranged it with your doctor or you may get an infection.

In some patients urinary retention is of a much more insidious nature. These patients often complain only of urinary frequency and urgency and it is not until they seek medical care that the true cause of their symptoms is discovered. In simplistic terms there are only two possible causes of urinary retention—either there is a blockage in the urethra or the bladder fails to contract during attempts to urinate. Urethral obstruction is very common in men, but very rare in women, unless they've had previous surgery on the bladder or urethra. In men obstruction is usually due to an enlarged prostate. An enlarged prostate may be caused by a benign growth—a natural consequence of aging called benign prostatic hyperplasia—or by a cancerous growth in the prostate. Another cause of urethral obstruction in men is urethral stricture. A urethral stricture is a scar in the wall of the urethra that causes a narrowing that is responsible for the blockage. The most common cause of urethral strictures in the United States is previous urethral surgery or instrumentation such as passage of a catheter or cystoscope. Less common causes include gonorrhea and fracture of the bones of the pelvis. Gonorrhea is a venereal disease that is often asymptomatic in women. During sexual intercourse, the gonococcal bacteria is transmitted from the woman to the man, and after a period of pain, burning, and urethral discharge, the man may develop a urethral stricture. Fractures of the pelvis are usually the result of automobile accidents or falls from great heights.

The other cause of urinary retention is weak or absent bladder contractions, which may be due to any neurologic condition that damages the nerves (such as spinal cord injury, herniated disc, or multiple sclerosis) or to an abnormality of the bladder muscle itself. In fact, overstretching of the bladder, as might occur during surgery or childbirth when the patient cannot feel bladder distension, can permanently damage the bladder and impair its ability to contract.

BLOODY URINE (HEMATURIA)

Blood in the urine is called *hematuria* (heem-a-tour-ia) and it is always abnormal (unless the urine was collected during menstruation and blood accidentally got into the urine sample). When there is so much bleeding that it is visible to the naked eye the proper term is *gross hematuria*. Bleeding that is only detected by looking at the urine under the microscope is called *microscopic hematuria*. Gross hematuria may manifest as pink, red, or burgundy-colored urine. When bleeding is severe, blood clots may be passed in the urine as well. Blood in the urine, whether gross or microscopic, should never be taken lightly. Overwhelmingly, the most common cause is just a simple bladder infection, but it may also be a sign of bladder cancer, kidney cancer, prostate cancer, and other serious conditions. This means that it should always be checked out by a doctor.

How should it be checked out? First, it needs to be established whether or not it is a sign of infection. This is done by obtaining a urine culture. Sometimes, though, patients may have a urinary infection *and* an underlying cancer, and it's important to be able to determine that with certainty. In general, if you do have a urinary tract infection and it's treated, the blood will go away on subsequent examinations and there is probably no need for further tests. However, if the blood does not go away, or if there wasn't an infection in the first place, it is necessary to check very carefully for the cause. Special urine tests called cytologies should be done to see if there are any cancer cells in the urine, and an imaging technique should be done to visualize the kidneys to make sure there are no stones or tumors. This can be a kidney X ray (an intravenous pyelogram), a CAT scan of the kidneys, or in some instances, an MRI (magnetic resonance image). In addition, cystoscopy (visual examination of the bladder with an cystoscope) should also be done. These topics are all discussed in more detail in Chapter 4. But remember, blood in the urine should always be checked by a doctor.

What kind of doctor?

The first time it's fine to see a primary care doctor, a general practitioner, an internist, or a gynecologist. If it's definitely proven to be sign of a urinary tract infection, and after treatment another urine test detects no blood, you're fine. If the blood does not go away, or if there is no infection, or if you get recurring episodes of blood in the urine, you should see a urologist.

CONCLUSION

The bladder is an unreliable witness. It has only a limited way of letting you know that it is not working properly or that it is diseased. There are hundreds of diseases and conditions that may affect the bladder, but no matter what is wrong, there are only five sets of symptoms that you can feel: (1) urinary frequency, urgency, and nocturia; (2) loss of urinary control (urinary incontinence); (3) pain; (4) difficulty passing urine, or the inability to urinate at all (urinary retention); and (5) blood in the urine (hematuria).

4

How to Determine the Cause of Bladder Symptoms

You get a sudden, severe urge to urinate and rush to the bathroom, but when you get there you manage to force out only a few drops of urine while your insides feel like they are on fire. Fifteen minutes later the same thing happens again, and then again and again. With symptoms of such intensity, only a stoic would fail to see a doctor. But what about the person who has a single episode of bloody urine, or the person who notices a gradual onset of difficulty initiating urination, or the person who is in the bathroom every hour around the clock, or the person who is incontinent and thinks there is nothing that can be done. All of these people should see a doctor and in almost every instance there will be an appropriate therapy that is likely to cure the condition.

WHEN TO SEE THE DOCTOR

There are two reasons to see a doctor for urinary bladder symptoms (or for that matter any other symptoms). The first, and foremost, reason is to determine whether or not your symptoms are the sign of a serious condition that, if undiagnosed, unrecognized, or untreated could go on to cause serious medical complications or even death. Untreated bladder, kidney, and prostate cancer can and do cause death, and, as is the case with most cancers, the key to cure is early diagnosis and treatment. Kidney stones can destroy kidneys; fortunately they usually cause a great deal of pain so an early diagnosis is usually obvious. Damage to the nerves of the bladder can also destroy kidneys, but this often causes no pain and minimal symptoms.

For that reason, early diagnosis is much more difficult, and for many patients the condition is not diagnosed until the kidneys are already damaged.

The second reason to see a doctor is because your symptoms bother you and you want them treated. For example, if you are incontinent, you are wetting your pants, which is causing you embarrassment and interfering with your job and your sex life. In short, incontinence is ruining your life. Or you urinate every half hour both day and night because it hurts too much if you don't urinate, so you end up planning your entire day around the availability of a bathroom. Or you're so frightened that you won't be able to urinate at all that you spend all of your time in the bathroom trying to go.

Most people see their physician when they have these kinds of symptoms because they are so overwhelmed by them that they have little choice . . . unless they think it's hopeless or they're too embarrassed. Hopeless because they've seen a doctor before and gotten no help, or because they've heard or read that "there's nothing that can be done," or "it's all in your head," or it's too expensive or too time consuming. Embarrassed because they think that they are unique, that no one else has ever had this problem, that it's a sign of inferiority or shame or disgust. Embarrassed because they think that they smell or they feel dirty.

So when should you go to the doctor? You go to the doctor whenever you have a persistent symptom that you want treated because it bothers you—you are the judge. From a medical viewpoint no one is quite so unique as he or she thinks. No matter what your symptoms are, someone else has had those same symptoms before and almost surely there is an effective way to diagnose and treat the condition. Most likely, your doctor has seen these symptoms many times before. If he or she has not seen them before, you might get another opinion from a doctor who is more experienced with your particular symptoms.

How do I know if my doctor is experienced with my symptoms?

Ask him!

There are certain symptoms that serve as a warning signal, a clue that there might be a more serious condition that needs evaluation and treatment even if you don't think the symptoms are so bad. These are so important that whenever they occur you should see a physician who is an expert at diagnosis and treatment. In most instances that physician is one who specializes in urinary bladder disorders. This specialty of medicine is called urology and the specialist is called a urologist. The symptoms that demand immediate attention are very few:

1. Bloody Urine (hematuria). This may manifest as bright red bloody urine and blood clots (as if you cut yourself) or may be

more subtle. The urine may be blood tinged, or burgundy, rose, or salmon colored. Many times the blood is only visible under the microscope when a urinalysis is performed either because you have other urinary symptoms or as part of a routine medical checkup.

No matter what the circumstances, blood in the urine (with the exception of menstrual blood) demands prompt attention. The most common cause of hematuria is a urinary tract infection, which generally responds quite well to antibiotics. However, hematuria may also be the only sign of serious conditions such as bladder, prostate, and kidney tumors as well as bladder and kidney stones.

2. Urinary frequency, urgency, and pain. When the symptoms are acute (they come on suddenly and you've never experienced them before) you should see a physician as soon as is reasonably convenient depending on the nature and severity of the symptoms. Obviously, if the symptoms are unbearable you should see a physician the same day. If they are more mild, the next available appointment within a few days is OK, especially since in some instances the symptoms are self-limited and will disappear by themselves. If the symptoms are of gradual onset and not too bothersome, an appointment within a month is probably appropriate.

The most common cause of these symptoms is a urinary tract infection; however, they may also be caused by more serious bladder, prostate, or kidney conditions.

WHAT DOCTORS DO

To obtain a diagnosis, the physician must take a detailed medical history, perform a relevant physical examination, obtain appropriate laboratory tests, and, in selected cases, obtain a voiding diary and pad test, appropriate X rays, urodynamic tests, and cystoscopy. All of these words are explained in the glossary and later in this chapter.

History

It is axiomatic that all diagnosis begins with a detailed analysis of your current symptoms. In addition, your doctor should ask about your previous medical and family history. He or she should ascertain what medications you are currently taking, whether you have any allergies, and whether you've had previous surgery.

From a historical perspective it is important to understand the precise nature of your symptoms and, in particular, what symptoms are most distressing. Do you really want treatment or just reassurance that the symptoms are not indicative of a more serious underlying condition? How often do you urinate during the day and at night? Why do you void as often as you do? Is it because of a severe urge or is it merely out of convenience or an attempt to prevent incontinence?

Do you lose control of urination (incontinence)? How severe is the incontinence? Do you lose just a few drops or do you saturate your clothing? Do you wear protective pads? Do they become saturated? How often do you change them? Are you aware óf when and how you actually wet yourself or do you just find yourself wet? Do you get a sense of urgency first? If so, how long can you hold before you must get to the bathroom? Do you lose urine when you cough or sneeze or during aerobics or sex? If the incontinence is associated with stress, do you only lose urine for an instant during the stress or do you void uncontrollably? Is the incontinence positional? Does it ever occur when you are lying or sitting still?

Is there difficulty starting the urine steam? Do you have to push and strain to get started? Is the stream weak or interrupted? Have you ever been completely unable to urinate? Have you ever had to be catheterized?

The past medical history and review of symptoms should focus on detecting symptoms of neurologic conditions such as multiple sclerosis, spinal cord injury, myelodysplasia, diabetes, stroke, or Parkinson's disease. It is important that your doctor know about double vision, muscular weakness, paralysis or poor coordination, numbness, or tingling because any of these can be symptoms of previously undetected neurologic problems. Your physician should also determine whether you have ever had previous surgery for incontinence, "a dropped bladder," pelvic relaxation, or cancer of the rectum or uterus.

Although medications only rarely cause urinary bladder symptoms, you should tell your doctor what medicines you are taking. Certain drugs used to treat high blood pressure may interfere with the nervous control of the urinary sphincter and cause stress incontinence. The most common of these are called sympatholytic agents and include drugs such as clonidine (Catapres), prazocin (Minipres), terazocin (Hytrin), and doxazocin (Cardura). Other drugs, such as bethanechol (Urecholine or Duvoid), may stimulate the bladder to contract involuntarily and cause urge incontinence. Certain other drugs used to treat the common cold, hay fever, and depression may cause difficulty urinating. These include combinations of medications that make the urethra contract, such as Sudafed, Ornade, etc., and medications that suppress bladder contractions, like tricyclic antidepressants such as imipramine (Tofranil). In either event, if the bladder fails to contract or if there is a blockage, difficulty urinating or even complete urinary retention may occur.

Voiding Diary

In order to document the nature and severity of bladder symptoms a voiding diary is indispensable. You'll be asked to complete this diary for a single representative 24-hour period. You will be given a printed diary form to be filled in each time you urinate. There are a number of different kinds of diaries depending on the specific nature of your symptoms, but certain features are common to all. The most important things to record are the time and volume of each urination and any symptoms that you associate with your condition. A sample diary is depicted in Figure 1.

This diary is used by people who complain of incontinence. Here's how it works. You record the time you first get an urge to urinate in the

NAME:_____   DATE:_____

TIME OF URGE TO VOID	STRENGTH OF PAIN OR URGE	TIME OF ACTUAL VOID	VOIDED VOLUME	INCONTINENCE (S, U OR W) see below	AMOUNT OF LEAKAGE (LARGE=L, MEDIUM=M, SMALL=S)
1.					
2.					
3.					
4.					
5.					
6.					
7.					
8.					
9.					
10.					
11.					
12.					
13.					
14.					
15.					
16.					
17.					

Urgency is the feeling that you have to urinate badly.

Incontinence is the loss of urine control before reaching the bathroom.
S = Stress Incontinence is wetting or leakage at times of coughing, sneezing, or with physical activity, etc.
U = Urge Incontinence is wetting or leakage because of urgency.
W = Unaware Incontinence is wetting without conscious awareness of when it happens.

Figure 1. Typical voiding diary.

first column. In the second column, you record the strength of the urge. For example, if you urinate as you are about to leave the house because you are afraid that you might get a severe urge on the ride to work, that would be a zero. On the other hand, if you have to stop the car to run to a gas station bathroom and leak a few drops on the way, that would be a ten. In the third column you record the actual time of urination. In the fourth column you record the actual amount (volume) that you void each time. This may be accomplished by urinating into a measuring cup that you keep in the bathroom or by carrying a supply of disposable coffee cups with you (you must first measure the volume that the coffee cup holds). In the last two columns, if incontinence has occurred, you record the time and estimated amount of urinary leakage as well as the circumstances during which the leakage occurred.

Pad Test

For people with urinary incontinence, a pad test is very useful. For a single 24-hour period, you wear protective pads, and change them as often as necessary. Each pad is placed in a plastic bag and brought to the doctor's office the next day. The pads are weighed, which allows the doctor to estimate the amount of urinary loss. Alternatively, you may be asked to take a pill that colors the urine orange or blue, and the doctor may merely inspect the pads and estimate the severity of urinary loss.

Physical Examination

The purpose of the physical examination is twofold. First, it is necessary to exclude anatomic and neurologic findings that might contribute to urinary incontinence. Second, the specific cause of the incontinence should be identified by visualizing the urinary loss. The means by which this is accomplished will be discussed in detail in the section entitled "Eyeball Urodynamics."

The physical examination begins with the first encounter between the doctor and patient. The doctor notices your overall appearance and physical characteristics when you first walk into the office. A slight limp or lack of coordination, an unusual speech pattern, facial asymmetry, or other physical characteristics, of which you might be completely unaware, may be the first sign of a subtle neurologic condition.

The examination should be conducted on an examining table with you lying on your back. All of your clothes from the waist down should be removed. Your doctor will palpate (feel) your abdomen with his fingers to search for previously undiagnosed tumors, hernias, or signs of an enlarged bladder. The doctor examines your rectum by passing a finger through the anal sphincter muscle into the rectum. While doing this, he or she notes the tone of the sphincter and determines whether or not you exhibit voluntary control. In order to do this, you will be asked to try to contract your anal sphincter muscle. Most people don't know what this means, so the doctor must be quite graphic. He or she might say, "pretend that you are in the middle of urinating and you suddenly want to stop; you must squeeze down around my finger," or "if you were afraid that you might lose control of your bowels or pass gas when you didn't want to, you would have to squeeze down around my finger." A lax or weakened anal sphincter or the inability to control the muscle are signs of neurologic damage. However, some people simply cannot understand the instructions and are unable to demonstrate their sphincter control to the doctor even though it is completely normal.

Another means of evaluating neurologic function is to test for the bulbocavernosus reflex. It is performed by suddenly squeezing the tip of the penis in men or the clitoris in women and noting the reflex contraction of the anal sphincter muscle. The absence of this reflex in men suggests that there could be a neurologic problem. This reflex is only present in about 70% of women, so the absence of the reflex in women is not as significant as it is in men.

Rectal examination may also disclose the presence of tumors, hemorrhoids, anal fissures, and blood in the stool. In men, the prostate is palpated for signs of enlargement or tumor. In women, a vaginal examination is performed with both a full and empty bladder.

Urodynamic Evaluation

Urodynamics refers to one or more tests in a series that is designed to measure and record a number of parameters from the bladder, urethra, and rectum that provide diagnostic information about the function of these organs. The specific urodynamic tests include (1) cystometry, (2) uroflow, (3) urethral pressure studies, (4) sphincter electromyography, and (5) synchronous multichannel video-urodynamic studies. Each of these tests is explained in detail below. These tests are often indispensable for diagnosing the cause of bladder symptoms. The purpose of any urodynamic evaluation is to exactly reproduce the patient's bladder symptoms by filling the bladder with fluid (to mimic the action of urine coming into the bladder from the kidneys). While the bladder is being filled and during urinating or attempts to urinate, appropriate observations are made either by simply watching the patient or by X ray. Simultaneously, measurements are made of the pressure inside of the bladder, urethra, and rectum. In selected cases, the electrical activity of the sphincter muscle (sphincter EMG) is also recorded.

Bladder symptoms reproduced during urodynamic tests will help pinpoint any underlying abnormality. Urodynamic technique may vary from "eyeball urodynamics" to sophisticated studies that combine many of the tests simultaneously. The makeup of your particular examination will depend on a multitude of factors including your medical history, the outcome of prior diagnostic tests, the experience of the examiner, and the availability of urodynamic testing facilities. Sophisticated multichannel video-urodynamics offers the most comprehensive and precise means of arriving at the correct diagnosis, but these tests are available at only a few centers throughout the world.

Fortunately, many patients can be adequately diagnosed and treated with much simpler technology. However, there are certain circumstances when these sophisticated studies are necessary: (1) if you complain of incontinence, but the cause cannot be determined; (2) if you have previously undergone corrective surgery for incontinence; (3) if you've undergone radical pelvic surgery for colon cancer or cancer of the uterus, cervix, or vagina; (4) if you have a known or suspected neurologic condition such as multiple sclerosis, stroke, spina bifida, spinal cord injury, or Parkinson's disease; (5) if you have lower urinary tract symptoms that have not improved despite treatment; or (6) if you have difficulty voiding, incomplete bladder emptying, or inability to urinate at all and the diagnosis is not clear or you've failed other treatments.

In many women an accurate diagnosis may be attained by detailed history, physical examination, and a simpler, less expensive form of urodynamics that I call "eyeball urodynamics." Unfortunately, this technique is not very accurate in men and I don't recommend it for them.

Eyeball Urodynamics

"Eyeball urodynamics" is a method of obtaining important diagnostic information without using any electronic equipment. The test is performed by inserting a catheter, a small, flexible tube, through the urethra and into your bladder. Some women feel a little discomfort on passage of the catheter, but it is almost never painful. Just prior to the examination you'll be asked to urinate and when the catheter is inserted the postvoid residual urine (the amount of urine remaining in the bladder after normal urination) is measured. After the bladder has been emptied, a syringe is

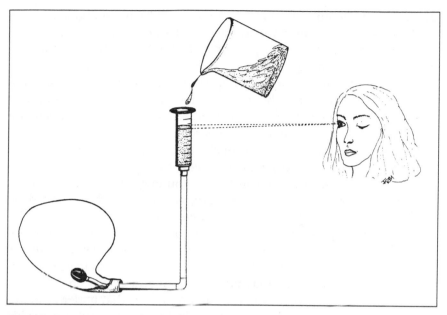

Figure 2. Eyeball urodynamics. Your bladder is filled with a fluid through a catheter. As the bladder is filled, you will be asked to report what you feel to your doctor. He or she will make observations and measurements that help diagnose the cause of your symptoms.

connected to the end of the catheter and saline (salt water that mimics the chemical contents of body fluids) or water is poured in through the open end of the syringe and allowed to drip into the bladder by gravity (Figure 2). As the water level in the syringe falls, the examiner can estimate the pressure inside the bladder simply by noting the change in the height of the water level in the syringe. As the bladder fills the patients is instructed neither to urinate nor to inhibit urination. Rather she is asked simply to report her sensations to the examiner. As soon as a change in pressure is noted, the examiner should question the patient to determine if she is aware of any symptom, such as the urge to urinate. In most instances the cause of a rise in bladder pressure will be obvious, but if it is in doubt, formal cystometry (discussed below) with rectal pressure monitoring is necessary. In many instances, the cause of your incontinence will be easily detected during this examination as an involuntary contraction of the bladder, which causes you to urinate uncontrollably around the catheter.

When your bladder has been filled until you feel a comfortable fullness, the catheter is removed (this is not a test to see how much fluid you can hold or how much the doctor can force in). Then the vagina is examined for signs of a prolapsed (dropped) bladder (cystocele) or uterus. These are usually obvious to your doctor as bulges in the vaginal wall. You'll be asked to cough and bear down in order to determine whether that causes incontinence. If you complain of urinary incontinence, but it has not been demonstrated by this examination, the examination may be repeated in the standing position. Although this may be embarrassing for you, it is a necessary part of the examination. It is best performed by having you stand with one foot on a small stool. Your doctor sits beside you and performs a vaginal examination while you cough and strain. If the incontinence still remains undemonstrable, you might be given a prescription for a urinary dye, such as Pyridium, which stains the urine a deep orange. You'll be asked to wear incontinence pads and tampons and instructed to bring the stained pads and tampons with you to the next office visit. The amount and location of the staining may help to determine the site and degree of urinary loss. In addition, you will probably need to undergo more sophisticated urodynamic studies and cystoscopy (looking into the bladder). It is very important to emphasize that under ordinary circumstances, no patient should undergo invasive surgery or irreversible treatment until the cause of the incontinence has been clearly demonstrated.

Cystometry

Cystometry is performed by filling the bladder through a catheter and measuring your bladder pressure, sensations, and the amount of fluid that is instilled. In fact, it is identical to eyeball urodynamics except that it is usually performed with a machine called a cystometer, which electronically measures bladder pressure and produces a graph called a cystometrogram. The main purpose of cystometry is to determine whether or not the bladder contracts involuntarily to cause incontinence and whether bladder filling causes pain or discomfort.

Uroflow

The assessment of urinary flow rate (uroflow) is a noninvasive, simple, inexpensive, and cost-effective screening procedure that provides important information about how well the bladder and urethra work together. All you do is stand or sit at a special urinal and urinate into a funnel. The rate of urinary flow and the amount that you void is calculated electronically and displayed on a graph. If the flow is normal, the chances are that there is no blockage in the urethra. However, if the flow is low, more testing will be needed to determine whether it is due to an obstruction (like a blockage from the prostate) or a weak bladder. In order to make the distinction between a blockage and a weak bladder, it is necessary to measure uroflow and bladder pressure simultaneously.

Bladder (Detrusor) Pressure/Uroflow Studies

Measuring bladder (detrusor) pressure and uroflow simultaneously is the only way of determining whether a low flow is due to a weak bladder or a urethral blockage. To do this test, it is necessary to urinate with a small catheter in the urethra so that bladder pressure can be measured at the same time as the urinary flow rate is measured. If the bladder contracts strongly, but the flow is weak, then there is a blockage. If the bladder contracts weakly, or not at all, and the flow is low, then the bladder itself is weakened. Of course, it is possible to have both a weak bladder and blockage in the urethra.

Sphincter Electromyography

Sphincter electromyography is an examination of the electric potentials generated by the muscle of the urethral sphincter.

What does that mean, electric potentials generated by the muscle? Am I plugged in, or what? Is there actually electricity in my body?

When a muscle contracts, there is a sudden change in its chemistry. A lot of positively and negatively charged chemicals called ions change places. The net result is that an electric current is created, and this electric current can be measured as an electromyograph (EMG). When there is a lot of EMG activity, the muscle is contracting; when there is no activity, the muscle is relaxed. Sphincter electromyography may be performed by pasting small patches, identical to the ones used for an EKG, on either side of the rectum. This does not hurt or cause any discomfort at all; however, the EMG signal is not as accurate as when a needle electrode is used. A needle electrode is a tiny, thin needle that is inserted just above the rectum in men and next to the urethra in women. Passage of the needle is painful for most people. Accordingly, this kind of electromyography is rarely done, and when it is, it is done for the purpose of obtaining important information in people who are suspected of having serious neurologic problems.

Two general kinds of diagnostic information may be attained from the sphincter EMG. First, the overall activity of the muscle during bladder filling and bladder contraction can be assessed. Second, the actual wave form and other characteristics of the EMG signal give a lot of information about whether or not the nerves and muscles are normal. Sphincter electromyography is always performed in conjunction with cystometry and may be combined with other studies as well.

Synchronous Multichannel Video-Urodynamic Studies

Why must doctors use such big words? There must be another way of saying this.

Synchronous measurement means measuring more than one thing at the same time. For people with bladder problems, it's important to measure the pressure in the bladder, the pressure in the rectum, and the rate of urinary flow all at the same time. Multichannel means that each measurement is displayed on a separate region of a graph. Video refers to viewing an X-ray picture of the bladder and urethra at the same time that the measurements are being taken. I call it video-urodynamics. If you can think of a simpler way of saying this, please let me know.

There are important advantages to video-urodynamics compared to doing the individual tests one at a time. By simultaneously measuring multiple urodynamic variables one gains a better insight into the underlying abnormalities. Moreover, since all variables are visualized simultaneously, one can better appreciate their interrelationships and identify artifacts with ease.

The technique of video-urodynamics is similar to that of cystometry and eyeball urodynamics (see above), but a little more involved. You will first be examined while lying on your back with your knees in stirrups. The vaginal area in women or the penis in men is gently washed with antiseptic soap. A very small catheter is passed through the urethra into the bladder and the bladder is emptied. Another small catheter is passed into the rectum. The catheters are connected to electronic equipment that records the pressures inside the bladder, rectum, and urethra. The bladder is filled through the catheter with a liquid that can be seen by X ray (X-ray contrast material), and periodically X-ray images are recorded on videotape. As the bladder is being filled, your doctor is in constant communication with you. Since the purpose of the test is to reproduce your urinary symptoms, you will be frequently asked whether or not you feel the symptoms that brought you to the doctor's office in the first place. If one of your complaints is incontinence, the doctor may ask you to bear down or cough to try to cause the incontinence. If your complaint is difficulty with urination or inability to urinate you will be asked to try to urinate. The measurements will usually provide information to pinpoint the cause of the problem.

The test sounds gruesome and you're probably concerned that it's painful. In women, passage of the catheter is rarely painful at all; in men, a small amount of discomfort is generally felt. Nevertheless, if you're experiencing more discomfort than you're comfortable with, tell the doctor and he or she may terminate the test. In some cases a local anesthetic will be used to pass the catheter.

Your doctor and his or her staff should understand your concerns about privacy and modesty and try to make things as comfortable for you as possible. They understand that it is often not possible to be relaxed in such bizarre circumstances (Figure 3). Nevertheless, worldwide, hundreds

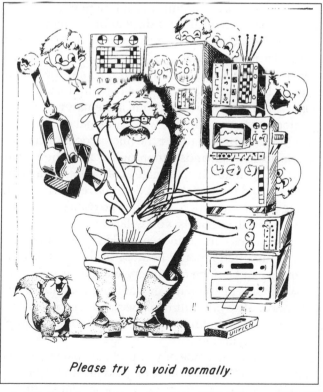

Please try to void normally.

Figure 3. Video-urodynamic study. Courtesy of J. G. Blaivas and Bob Ullrich.

of thousands of people have been evaluated with these tests and it's been repeatedly shown that an accurate diagnosis can be achieved in the vast majority of patients.

There are a few possible complications from the test: (1) urinary tract infection, (2) painful or frequent urination, (3) difficulty urinating or inability to urinate at all, and (4) blood in the urine (hematuria). These complications are rare, occurring in less than 5% of patients. Most of the patients who experience these complications have preexisting conditions that make a complication much more likely to occur. If you have a preexisting condition, appropriate precautions to prevent a complication will be taken.

CONCLUSION

Urinary symptoms are of concern for two reasons. First, the symptoms themselves may be bothersome and interfere with your day-to-day functioning. They may cause pain and discomfort, so they need treatment in their own right. Second, the symptoms, even if not terribly bothersome, may signal a more serious underlying condition that, if not diagnosed and treated, could impair your health. Accordingly, any persistent urinary symptoms should be thoroughly evaluated by your doctor.

The most serious bladder symptom is hematuria (bloody urine). Whether it's blood that you can see with your naked eye (gross hematuria) or blood that is only seen under the microscope (microscopic hematuria), hematuria always demands a thorough examination by a urologist. Urinary retention—the inability to urinate at all—also always requires immediate evaluation and treatment, but I don't have to tell you that. If you experience acute urinary retention, you have no choice; it hurts too much. So it is with pain as well; if it hurts, you will come.

The other symptoms—incontinence, difficulty urinating, urinary frequency, etc.—are too often ignored because of the mistaken impression that either nothing can be done or surgery will be necessary. For people with bladder symptoms of any kind, evaluation by a knowledgeable professional will almost always result in an accurate diagnosis and effective treatment. A knowledgeable professional is, more often than not, a specialist—a urologist or gynecologist.

Now a word of caution. Some of you probably belong to health maintenance organizations (HMOs) or other prepaid health plans. These health care providers discourage patients from seeing specialists until they have been screened by a general practitioner or family practice physician. The logic behind this is simple. Specialists are more expensive than primary care doctors or nurse practitioners. Moreover, in most instances, the initial symptoms of any condition are either cured or subside by themselves with minimal intervention from the medical profession. That's fine if you go to the doctor and your symptoms are cured. But if they're not cured, if they persist or get worse, it's time to see a specialist and it may be time to have one of these tests.

5

Urinary Frequency, Urgency, and Urge Incontinence

INTRODUCTION

Urinary frequency, urgency, and urge incontinence are a group of symptoms each of which may occur alone or, more commonly, in combination with one another. Urinary frequency is simply defined as the need to urinate more often than normal. There are no exact normal numbers, although most people urinate about six to eight times a day. When we ask patients how often they normally urinate, the most common answer is, "it varies." For any one person, the frequency of urination *is* very variable, depending on the many factors which are discussed in Chapter 1.

Some people are quite comfortable urinating once every hour or two; others find it very distressing to interrupt their activities to go to the bathroom more than three or four times a day. From *your own* perspective, though, urinary frequency can be defined as urinating more often than *you* are comfortable with. If you used to void four times a day and now you void seven times a day, for *you*, that's urinary frequency.

The frequency of urination depends on two basic factors: how much urine your body makes and how much urine your bladder can comfortably hold before it signals the need to urinate. As we've just noted, the amount of urine that the kidneys make is dependent primarily on how much you eat and drink. The more you eat and drink, the more urine your kidneys produce. The amount of urine that your bladder can comfortably hold is also dependent on a number of factors. Bladder infection (cystitis), other inflammations of the bladder, and bladder tumors greatly reduce the volume that the bladder can comfortably hold. Women urinate more often during pregnancy because their bladders don't hold as much, probably because of the weight of the uterus pushing on the bladder. Other conditions such as radiation treatments to the lower abdomen, multiple operations on the bladder, and bladder hypersensitivity also greatly reduce the capacity of the bladder. Neurologic disorders such as multiple sclerosis, stroke, and spinal cord injury also reduce the capacity of the bladder. No matter what the original cause, if your bladder capacity becomes reduced, it tends to stay that way, like a bad habit, unless you undergo treatment.

Urinary urgency is the feeling that urination is imminent, that it cannot be postponed for more than a matter of moments. When you get the feeling of urinary urgency, you stop what you are doing and rush to the bathroom, either because of severe discomfort or a feeling that you will lose control and wet yourself. Urinary urgency is different from the normal urge to urinate. The normal urge is felt as a vague sensation of fullness in the lower abdomen or as a tingly or sharp sensation at the tip of the penis in men or in the urethra in women. Urge incontinence is a sudden loss of urinary control, associated with the sensation of urgency. In some instances, a person with urge incontinence gets a sudden urge and is able momentarily to prevent the leakage. He or she just barely makes it to the bathroom, but loses control once there. In more severe cases, there may be no more than a second's warning of urgency before the person simply loses control of his or her bladder. Table 1 lists the most common causes of urinary frequency, urgency, and urge incontinence.

Bladder Inflammation (Cystitis)

Cystitis is an inflammation of the bladder. The most common cause of cystitis is *infection* with bacteria, but in some rare cases there may be infections due to tuberculosis, fungus, and other kinds of microorganisms. When bacterial cystitis is the cause, the symptoms almost always subside once the infection is treated with the proper antibiotic. However, there are a number of kinds of cystitis that are not due to infection and cannot be treated with antibiotics. These include inflammation of the bladder due to radiation treatment and certain kinds of chemotherapy, such as the drug cyclophosphamide (Cytoxan) used to treat cancer. Stress and anxiety do not cause cystitis, but cystitis can make you more stressed and anxious. In Chapter 6 you will learn all about the different kinds of cystitis and how they are diagnosed and treated.

Table 1. Causes of Urinary Frequency, Urgency, and Urge Incontinence

Small-capacity bladder (the bladder doesn't hold enough urine)
1. Bladder inflammation (cystitis)
2. Bladder hypersensitivity (interstitial cystitis, prostatitis)
3. Bladder overactivity (involuntary contractions of the bladder)
   A. Detrusor instability (involuntary contractions of the bladder due to nonneurologic conditions)
      1. Urethral obstruction (enlarged prostate, urethral scars)
      2. Sphincteric incontinence (in women)
      3. Bladder stones or foreign body or prostate cancer
      4. Bladder or prostate cancer
   B. Detrusor hyperreflexia (involuntary contractions of the bladder due to neurologic conditions)
      1. Multiple sclerosis
      2. Stroke
      3. Parkinson's disease
      4. Spinal cord injury
      5. Spina bifida (myelodysplasia)
Polyuria (the kidneys make too much urine)
1. Habit
2. Diabetes mellitus (abnormality of insulin regulation)
3. Diabetes insipidus (abnormality of regulation of urine by kidneys)
   A. Nephrogenic (kidney abnormalities)
      1. Diseases that affect the kidney (sarcoidosis, polycystic kidneys, sickle cell anemia, kidney infections)
      2. Reaction to medications (lithium, demeclocycline, methoxyflurane)
      3. Hereditary
   B. Neurologic (traumatic head injuries, brain tumors, brain infections, brain aneurysms)
4. Excessive thirst
   A. Psychologic (schizophrenia, manic-depression)
   B. Neurologic (brain infections, multiple sclerosis)

Bladder Hypersensitivity (Interstitial Cystitis)

Normally, as the bladder fills with urine from the kidneys, there are no sensations at all until the bladder begins to get full, signaling the need to urinate. In patients with bladder hypersensitivity, bladder filling itself is uncomfortable and as capacity is reached it becomes painful. People with bladder hypersensitivity urinate frequently because it hurts if they do not. The cause of these painful bladder symptoms is not known, but intense research is underway looking into both diagnosis and treatment. It is important for people with painful bladder syndromes to undergo a proper evaluation to be sure that the symptoms are not being caused by infection or more serious conditions such as bladder or prostate cancer. (This topic is discussed in detail in Chapter 10.)

Bladder Overactivity (Involuntary Contractions of the Bladder)

In some people, the symptoms of urinary frequency, urgency, and urge incontinence are due to bladder overactivity. Bladder overactivity is a general term that means that the bladder contracts involuntarily. When an involuntary bladder contraction occurs, it usually signals the beginning of urination. If your sensations are normal, you feel this involuntary bladder contraction as an urge to urinate and immediately (either consciously or subconsciously) contract your sphincter. This stops the urination and makes the bladder stop contracting. You might then go to the bathroom and urinate, or you may delay urination until you feel another urge to urinate. If you are unable to stop the bladder contraction, you will lose control of urination.

There are many causes of involuntary bladder contractions, but they can be divided into two main groups depending on whether or not the underlying cause is due to an abnormality of the nerve supply (innervation) to the bladder. When there is an abnormality of innervation, the condition is called *detrusor hyperreflexia* and the person is said to have a neurogenic bladder (*detrusor* [dee-troo-sore] is the medical term for the muscle in the wall of the bladder). When there is not a neurologic cause of the involuntary bladder contractions, the condition is called *detrusor instability*. Detrusor instability is often associated with other conditions such as urethral obstruction, stress incontinence, infection, bladder and prostate cancer, and bladder stones. Most of the time, when these conditions are successfully treated detrusor overactivity subsides as well. When there is no obvious cause of detrusor overactivity, the cause is said to be idiopathic. *Idiopathic* is a fancy medical term that means "disease of unknown origin." A very common kind of idiopathic bladder overactivity is "garage door syndrome."

"Door Key" or "Garage Door Syndrome"

In many patients, urinary urgency and urge incontinence (due to detrusor instability) seem to be triggered by certain conditions, the most dramatic example of which is the "door key" or "garage door syndrome." In this situation, you feel perfectly normal, with no urge to urinate until your car pulls into the driveway and the garage door starts to go up or you put your key in the door lock. Then, suddenly, you get a severe urge to urinate and must rush to the bathroom. If you don't get there in time, you start to urinate without control. In some patients, only a drop or two of urine leaks out; others lose total control and completely wet themselves.

A more common scenario is the urge to void that many people experience when they are close to running water. Washing the dishes, washing your hands, or just hearing the sound of running water sends many normal people right to the bathroom. If you experience the urge to urinate when near running water, that is probably normal, but if you must stop what you are doing and rush to the bathroom or actually lose control along the way, that is abnormal.

What causes this to happen?

It's probably a conditioned reflex—a reflex that is gradually developed in the body by the frequent repetition of a specific stimulus. For example, if as a baby you burn your finger in a flame, the next time you feel the heat of a flame, you'll pull your finger away, even before it is burned. Eventually, you'll immediately pull your finger away every time you see a flame, even if you don't feel the heat. That's called a conditioned reflex.

I don't get it. Why would I get a sudden urge to urinate once I get to my front door?

Well, most people, if they get an urge to urinate while on a bus or in their car, will wait until they get home to urinate because it's more comfortable and they won't have to go looking for a strange bathroom. If that happens to you a lot, you subconsciously begin to associate putting the key in the lock with the urge to void and, eventually, it can happen uncontrollably.

TREATMENT

The most important aspect of treatment is to attain an accurate diagnosis and to eliminate the cause of your symptoms. When bacterial infection is the cause, treatment with culture-specific antibiotics is usually curative within 48 hours. If you have an infection and take antibiotics and the symptoms persist, you are either (1) not taking the medicine properly, (2) the medicine is the wrong one for that infection, or (3) the infection was not the only cause of the symptoms. The medicine could be the wrong medicine for your infection if the bacteria are resistant to the antibiotic or if the infection was caused by a virus or other microorganism for which the antibiotic is ineffective.

When bladder or prostate cancer is the cause, cure of the cancer usually results in cure of the symptoms. Bladder stones are usually caused by another underlying abnormality such as prostatic obstruction or retained sutures from previous surgeries. Very often, even after the stones are removed, it is necessary to treat the condition that caused the stones in the first place.

Radiation cystitis, cystitis due to chemotherapy, and interstitial cystitis require specialized treatment. This is discussed in detail in Chapters 9 and 10.

TREATMENT OF INVOLUNTARY BLADDER CONTRACTIONS

There are three basic treatments for involuntary bladder contractions: (1) treating the underlying (remediable) cause, (2) behavior modification, and (3) medications. Only when these treatments fail is it necessary to go on to more invasive therapies.

Treatment of Remediable Conditions

A remediable condition is one in which successful treatment makes the symptoms go away. For example, if you have burning when you urinate and you have an infection, cure of the infection makes the burning go away. The infection was a remediable condition. Treatment of the underlying cause of involuntary bladder contractions makes the most sense. Unfortunately, most people do not have a remediable underlying cause, and even when they do, treatment may require major surgery, which you might not want to undergo. After infection, the most common remediable causes of involuntary bladder contractions are prostatic obstruction in men and stress incontinence in women. Relieving the obstruction (as discussed in Chapters 11 and 12) and treating stress incontinence (Chapter 8) are the most effective ways of treating involuntary bladder contractions. Women, too, may have urethral obstruction causing involuntary bladder contractions, but this is almost always due to scarring from prior surgery, and when this is the case, further surgery is necessary to correct the problem. Rarely, involuntary bladder contractions may be the first sign of bladder cancer.

Behavior Modification

Behavior modification deals with observable and measurable behaviors that actually cause your symptoms by teaching you to change those behaviors so that you no longer have symptoms. Behavior modification is an effective form of treatment for the symptoms of urinary frequency, urgency, and urge incontinence. It is intended to treat your symptoms by "teaching" you to regain control of your bladder and sphincter. Some of the principles are quite simple. For example, the less fluid you drink, the less urine your body makes, and the less chance there is for incontinence. Other principles are much more complex and require that you keep a diary to track the complex interactions between you and the many things that occur in your day-to-day life that might influence your symptoms. Behavioral treatment usually consists of eight to twelve individual sessions with a behavioral therapist. The eight- to twelve-week period is an intensive bladder-retraining program that requires considerable expense of time and effort on the part of the patient and the therapist. Each week a voiding diary is kept by the patient (see Figure 1, Chapter 4). The diary consists of a number of notations including the time and amount of each urination (you need to measure the amount that you void), the time and nature of any incontinent episodes, and situational events surrounding the act of incontinence. In addition, you will be taught techniques for contracting the pelvic muscle that help to abort involuntary detrusor contractions. When there is associated bladder pain and stress, stress relaxation techniques are also taught. The muscle-contracting techniques are similar to Kegel exercises (see Chapter 8). In the middle of urinating, try to stop; that's the simplest way of learning how to contract the proper muscles. If you can't do that, you may need to be instructed in using biofeedback techniques. There are a number of stress relaxation techniques available, most of which require you to close your eyes, breathe deeply, and use different kinds of imagery. The best way to incorporate these into your treatment is through the process of behavioral modification with a properly trained therapist.

Behavior modification is effective in the great majority of patients and can even be used when there is an underlying condition causing the symptoms that cannot be effectively treated. For example, it has proven quite useful in patients with involuntary bladder contractions from such diverse conditions as multiple sclerosis, prostatic obstruction, and Parkinson's disease. There are two necessary ingredients for successful behavior modification: a motivated patient and a competent behavioral therapist. Unfortunately, there is currently a dearth of both. Most patients would rather take a pill, or even have an operation, than do behavior modification, and, sadly, there are not very many well-trained, competent behavioral therapists. Two pioneer behavioral therapists in the United States are Kathryn Burgio and Susan Blaivas (who happens to be my wife). I know both to be knowledgeable, practical, and empathic clinicians who rou-

COLLEGE OF THE SEQUOIAS
LIBRARY

tinely obtain excellent results treating even the most difficult bladder problems. For clinicians with such expertise, a motivated patient is the best insurance for a successful outcome.

Medications

There are two main kinds of medications that are used to treat involuntary bladder contractions: anticholinergics (ant-eye-kol-in-erj-ik) and tricyclic antidepressants. These drugs may be used singly or in combination with one another. Both types of medications work by interfering with the nerve impulses that make the bladder contract. With all of these medications, it is best to start at a low dose and gradually increase the medication over a period of days to weeks until you either have achieved the desired results or are experiencing side effects from the medication that prevent you from continuing to take it. This process is called dose titration. The time interval between doses depends on the half-life of the medicine. The half-life refers to how fast the active ingredient(s) is eliminated from the bloodstream. If the half-life is four hours, then four hours after taking the drug, only half is left in the bloodstream. If you do not take another dose of the medication, it will no longer exert its beneficial effect. The actual blood level that is necessary to prevent symptoms varies greatly, but since side effects are also related to the blood level, you may prefer to take this kind of medication only as needed. For example, you may take such a medication just as you are going to the movies, knowing that its effects will last about four hours. When you get home and are near a bathroom, you may prefer simply to urinate as soon as you get the urge rather than put up with side effects.

Some medications, though, build up a blood level. This means that not all of the medication is eliminated from the bloodstream and, with each successive dose, a little more remains until eventually, you take just enough medication to replace what is lost each day. Once you reach this level, you have a therapeutic blood level, which means that the medication is active all the time, 24 hours a day. But remember, not only do you receive the beneficial effects of the medication all the time, you may also experience the side effects.

Anticholinergics and Antispasmodics

Anticholinergics are medications that block the action of acetylcholine, the chemical messenger (a neurotransmitter) that stimulates the bladder to contract. Anticholinergic medications are used to stop involuntary bladder contractions. Antispasmodics also inhibit bladder contractions, but they act directly on the bladder muscle rather than by blocking a chemical messenger.

Oxybutynin (*Ditropan* and *Ditropan XL*). Oxybutynin comes in 2 forms, a short acting and a long acting. The short acting form is taken every 4–6 hours and gradually wears off after that. The short acting form is available both as generic and under the brand name Ditropan, which only need be taken once a day, is only available under the brand name Ditropan XL. Oxybutynin should be taken on an empty stomach with water, but if you develop nausea, it may be taken with meals or with a glass of milk. If symptoms persist on the starting dosage, you may double the dose after one week. You should return for an office visit within one to four weeks or so and your progress should be checked. Since the medication may weaken bladder contractions, it is important to check that you are urinating OK and that you empty the bladder satisfactorily. The best way to do this is to check the rate of urine flow (uroflow) by urinating into a flowmeter and measuring postvoid residual urine volume by ultrasound. Emptying the bladder satisfactorily does not necessarily mean that it is completely empty, although that is the ideal. There is no simple postvoid residual urine volume that is acceptable; rather, your doctor will need to make the judgment whether or not you are emptying satisfactorily based on many factors that he or she will have to take into consideration.

If your symptoms are sufficiently improved and you are urinating satisfactorily, the medication should be continued and you should be checked again in about three months. If the symptoms persist, further evaluation or treatment is needed.

The principal side effects include the following:

1. Dry mouth. This occurs in most patients. If your mouth does not get dry at all, it usually means that you are not taking enough medication. If the dry mouth becomes too uncomfortable, you may try chewing Biotene gum, which you can purchase in a pharmacy, to relieve the dry mouth symptoms.
2. Blurred vision. This side effect occurs in a very small percentage of patients but is usually disabling enough to warrant discontinuing the medicine. If it happens to you, stop the medication.
3. Rapid heart beat. This is usually felt as a "sudden shifting of gears" of the heart. The medicine should be stopped immediately and you should contact your physician.
4. Pain in the eye. *THIS IS A MEDICAL EMERGENCY.* You should discontinue the medication and contact your ophthalmologist or emergency room immediately. Pain in the eye could be a sign of a glaucoma attack. Glaucoma is high pressure inside of the eye. If

glaucoma persists and if not treated, it can cause blindness. This tragedy can be avoided by prompt treatment, which is usually nothing more than eye drops.

5. Urinary retention. In some patients, particularly those with prostatic obstruction, spinal cord injury, multiple sclerosis, or spina bifida, the medication is so effective that the patient is unable to urinate at all. In many people with neurologic conditions, such as spinal cord injury and multiple sclerosis, this is actually a desired effect and not really a side effect. The goal of therapy for them is to paralyze the bladder with medications and then empty the bladder with self intermittent catheterization. Intermittent catheterization is a means of emptying the bladder when you cannot urinate normally. It is performed by passing a small catheter into the bladder to empty the urine. It is usually done three to six times a day, depending on how much urine the bladder can safely hold. Intermittent catheterization is usually done by the patient and is called self intermittent catheterization, or SIC. Believe it or not, it is not painful; it can be done in just a few minutes and doesn't even need to be done with sterile technique. All you need is a catheter, which is used over and over again, and a little lubrication—no gloves, no tubes, no tape— it's really very simple. (This topic is discussed fully in Chapter 11.)

6. Constipation. Constipation may occur because the anticholinergic effect of the medication also inhibits intestinal contractions. The constipation can usually be adequately treated with cathartics.

7. Decreased sweating. Decreased sweating occurs because the sweat glands are inhibited by the anticholinergic action. For most people, this is not a problem, but patients with spinal cord injury and multiple sclerosis may not be able to cool down their bodies sufficiently in hot weather when taking anticholinergics.

8. Drowsiness.

Tolterodine (Detrol). Tolterodine is currently only available under the brand name Detrol. Its efficacy is about the same as Oxybutynin, but it has less side effects than the short acting version of Oxybutynin and about the same side effects as the long acting version.

Other Anticholinergics. The medications listed below work in a similar fashion to oxybutynin and have similar side effects. They will be described briefly, pointing out the major differences and usual dosages. Of course, you should never take these medications unless they have been prescribed by your physician; without proper supervision, they can be dangerous.

- *Propantheline* (ProBanthine). The usual starting dose is 7.5–15 mg four times a day, but some patients require as much as 30–60 mg three or four times a day.

- *Dicyclomine* (Bentyl). The starting dose is 20–40 mg four times a day.
- *Hyoscyamine.* There are a number of different formulations of hyoscyamine:

    Cystospaz. Starting dose is 1–2 tabs four times a day. It also comes in a sustained-release capsule called Cystospaz M. The starting dose is 1–2 tabs two times a day.

    Levsin. The usual dosage is 1–2 tabs every four hours. It also comes in a liquid form that can be taken at a dose of 1–2 tsp. every four hours as needed.

    Levsin SL (SL stands for sublingual). This medication is allowed to dissolve under your tongue. The usage dosage is 1–2 tabs every four hours.

    Levsinex timecaps. The usual dosage is 1–2 tabs every twelve hours as needed.

Fluvoxate (Urispas).   This drug is an antispasmotic. The starting dose is 100–200 mg four times a day.

Tricyclic Antidepressants

Imipramine (Tofranil).   Imipramine is usually begun at a dosage of 25 mg. It is given once a day, usually at bedtime. The medicine is increased by 25 mg per dose at weekly intervals up to maximum of approximately 150 mg per day. You will likely be told to return for an office visit at the end of four weeks and your progress will be evaluated in an identical fashion as for oxybutynin. The side effects and precautions are the same as for oxybutynin with several exceptions:

1. It should be used with caution in people with heart or thyroid disease because it can cause cardiac irregularities.
2. It should not be used at all if you are taking certain antidepressants called monoamine oxidase inhibitors (Nardil, Parnate) because it can cause serious heart problems.
3. In certain people, if discontinued suddenly, imipramine may cause mental depression. Accordingly, the dose should be cut down gradually under the supervision of your doctor.
4. In young children, accidental ingestion of imipramine can be fatal, so be sure that it is kept in tamper-proof containers out of the reach of children.

Because of all of these concerns, you should never take imipramine (or any other prescription drug for that matter) unless your doctor prescribes it. And, above all, you should always inform all of your physicians that you are taking imipramine so that they will be sure not to prescribe a medicine with which it interacts.

Biofeedback

Biofeedback is a technique designed to help you strengthen and gain control over your sphincter and gain control over your bladder. Biofeedback may be used alone or in combination with behavior modification and electrical stimulation. When used to treat urge incontinence, the best results are attained when it is combined with behavior modification. In this program, the purpose of biofeedback is to teach you how to contract your sphincter, which you do naturally each time you get a sudden urge to urinate. If you are successful, the sphincter contraction serves two purposes: It keeps urine from leaking out during an involuntary bladder contraction, and it activates a neurologic reflex that shuts off the bladder contraction.

The technique of biofeedback is as follows. A small balloonlike device is gently inserted into the vagina or rectum. You are instructed how to contract the sphincter muscles and the strength and duration of each muscle contraction are displayed on a screen as a graph or as blinking lights, or they may be signaled as a buzzing noise that increases in volume as the contraction increases in strength.

Biofeedback sessions are usually scheduled once a week. Based on the progress that you make each week, an exercise program is planned for the following week. The overall success rate for this treatment has not been determined. It seems to help many patients and some appear to be cured. There have not been any reported complications from this form of treatment.

Electrical Stimulation

Electrical stimulation of the sphincter muscle has been advocated by some as a method of treatment for urinary incontinence. The theory behind this treatment is that by stimulating the muscle to contract, it will strengthen the muscle, increase its tone, and through a negative feedback system, inhibit the bladder from contracting, much in the same way biofeedback does. Electrical stimulation is performed by placing a stimulation electrode either in or near the vagina or rectum or beneath the scrotum. The electrode may be a surface patch, like an EKG electrode, held in place with adhesive, or it may be shaped like a balloon (for the vagina) or an hourglass) for the rectum. Insertion of these electrodes is not painful at all, and there is no pain (or danger) during stimulation. The stimulation sessions are usually scheduled at weekly or biweekly intervals. In some instances, home stimulation units may be rented.

Absorbent Pads and Other Forms of Protection

There is a large selection of absorbent pads, panty liners, and adult diapers for both men and women that can be utilized to manage incontinence and prevent wetting of underwear and outer clothes. A complete list of current products are available in a number of different catalogues. The most user-friendly and extensive catalogue is the one published by The National Association for Continence, whose address is listed in Appendix B.

Surgical Treatment

Surgical treatment of urge incontinence should be considered only if you have persistent symptoms that have not responded to any of the more conservative forms of therapy. From a theoretical standpoint, there are two possible surgical interventions that could alleviate the problem of involuntary detrusor contractions. The nerve supply to the bladder could be altered by cutting or destroying the nerve endings so that the signals for bladder contraction would no longer be transmitted, or the bladder could be surgically altered so that it no longer contracts. Although there have been a number of surgical procedures that are designed to interfere with the nerve supply, none has met with widespread approval, and at this point in time I would not recommend any of them. The only technique that I have found to be efficacious is augmentation cystoplasty.

Augmentation Cystoplasty

Augmentation cystoplasty is a major operation in which part of the intestine is disconnected from the rest of the intestine and added on to the bladder. The purpose of the operation is to greatly increase the capacity of the bladder (increase the volume of urine that the bladder can hold before you urinate) and to prevent the bladder from contracting involuntarily. The success rate of the operation is in excess of 90% *but* many patients are unable to urinate naturally afterwards and must resort to intermittent self-catheterization.

As you might imagine, the decision to perform this operation should not be taken lightly. It is reserved for patients with symptoms of urinary frequency, urgency, or incontinence in whom all simpler forms of treatment have proven ineffective. Inasmuch as the intestines are going to be used in surgery, it is necessary for a thorough cleansing prior to surgery. For most patients, this cleansing can be accomplished on the day prior to the surgery. You are admitted to the hospital and over the course of approximately 12 hours drink a gallon of a cathartic fluid. This completely removes the solid waste products from the intestine. In addition, antibiotics are given by mouth to try to sterilize the bowel contents. Because so much fluid is lost during this "bowel prep," intravenous fluids are administered to replenish the lost fluid.

The actual surgery usually takes about three to five hours, but preoperative preparation in the operating room and postoperative recovery care take much longer. Accordingly, most patients leave their hospital room shortly after 7 AM and don't return to their hospital bed until late afternoon.

The operation is performed through a vertical incision extending from just above the belly button to just below the pubic hairline. At the time of surgery, a special catheter (suprapubic tube) is inserted into the bladder and comes out through the lower abdomen for the purpose of draining the urine. A second safety catheter, which also drains urine, is left in the urethra. These catheters stay in place approximately seven to ten days. Prior to their removal, a special X ray (cystogram) is obtained to be sure that the wound is healed. X-ray contrast fluid is instilled through the catheter and the process of bladder filling and emptying is monitored by fluoroscopy. If the X ray is normal, the catheter is removed and you are started on intermittent self-catheterization. Prior to each catheterization, you may attempt to urinate and if successful and the residual urine is low, it is possible that the intermittent catheterization may be discontinued. *However, at least 75% of patients undergoing this procedure require intermittent catheterization on a permanent basis.*

There are a number of potential complications, but the actual complication rate has been exceedingly low. The most common complication is wound infection, which is particularly common in patients with neurologic causes of their bladder condition such as multiple sclerosis, spinal cord injury, or spina bifida. It is also a particular problem in obese patients. The combination of obesity and paralysis from one of the above conditions raises the risk of wound infection after surgery, to about 25%.

The other postoperative complications are pretty much the same as for other major operations and generally pose little threat to one's health unless there are risk factors from other conditions such as serious heart or lung disease. The long-term consequences of augmentation cystoplasty are not well known. In general, when the bladder was a serious problem to start with (as in patients with spinal cord injury, spina bifida, and multiple sclerosis), the operation reverses most of the potentially serious conditions that might have ensued. However, as with any other intestinal surgery, there is the possibility of an intestinal obstruction or the formation of stones within the bladder itself, but to date these complications have been very infrequent. If the ureters were reimplanted during augmentation cystoplasty, it is possible that they could become obstructed or allow reflux of urine back up to the kidneys, but both of these conditions occur very infrequently.

There are reports in the medical literature of troublesome diarrhea occurring in 5–10% of patients, but this has not been my experience. In addition, there may be a lifelong need for vitamin B12 supplements after surgery, because some people are not able to absorb this vitamin properly afterward.

As you might imagine, not everyone will want to undergo such major surgery. For people who have already failed all reasonable conventional therapies and for others who don't even want to try them, experimental therapies might be considered.

Experimental Treatments

Medical treatment is in a perpetual state of evolution. Thanks to ongoing basic science and clinical research new therapies are developed and, when successful, they often replace existing treatments. Once a promising treatment has been shown to be potentially useful and safe in laboratory animals, further investigations are necessary to determine its overall efficacy and safety in humans. Human studies are very strictly regulated by the Federal Drug Administration (FDA).

At any given time, there are usually many different clinical research protocols involving new treatments. From my perspective, these protocols fall into one of three categories:

1. An entirely new treatment whose efficacy and safety are being tested in humans after animal studies have indicated that it will likely be both safe and efficacious. This is pure research and it may turn out that the treatment is of no use at all and may even be harmful. Experimental treatments, by definition, are risky.
2. A treatment that has been reasonably well evaluated for safety and efficacy and has been approved for use in other countries but has not been introduced into the USA. The FDA generally requires further studies in the USA to conform to its standards. Participation

in these kinds of studies may allow you to begin treatment with a new, more effective treatment before it is otherwise available. This kind of research usually has substantially less risk than the first kind.

3. An existing drug, already approved for use in the USA (because of efficacy and safety), is being tested because it shows promise for the treatment of another condition. In general, your doctor may offer you this treatment even if you don't want to participate in the research. Again, the drug's safety is by no means assured, but this poses the least risk of all.

Thus, even though all of these protocols are considered to be clinical research, some treatments are much more likely than others to be both safe and effective.

CONCLUSION

Urinary frequency (voiding too often) is probably the most common of all lower urinary tract symptoms. It may be caused by nothing more serious than drinking too much fluid or it may be the only initial sign of diabetes or a urinary tract infection. Simply put, if you urinate too much, it is either because you make too much urine or because your bladder doesn't hold enough.

Urinary urgency is a sudden feeling that you must urinate. It makes you stop what you are doing and look for a bathroom. Urge incontinence is the loss of urinary control because the urgency is so intense that you cannot hold back the urine. Urgency and urge incontinence are usually caused by involuntary contractions of the bladder. The most common cause is probably cystitis, but many other conditions commonly cause these symptoms. After urinary tract infection, the most common causes include an enlarged prostate in men and sphincteric incontinence in women, but in many women the cause is unknown. Occasionally, more serious conditions such as bladder or prostate cancer may present as urinary urgency and/or urge incontinence. Other causes of urinary frequency and urgency include interstitial and other rare forms of cystitis.

It is generally not possible to determine the cause of any of these symptoms without getting a proper medical evaluation. However, once you've seen a physician who is proficient at evaluating and treating these conditions, it is usually possible to attain an accurate diagnosis, and treatment will likely cure your symptoms.

6

Nocturia

Nocturia, derived from the Latin *noct,* night, and *uria,* urine, literally means urinating at night, but in its common usage, it means being awakened at night to urinate. Normally, most people sleep through the night or get up once or maybe twice to urinate. Getting up more than twice to urinate after you have gone to sleep for the night is considered to be abnormal. As a symptom, nocturia does not necessarily need treatment, but it is important to determine that the underlying cause of nocturia is not a more serious condition that requires treatment.

If your kidneys make more urine than your bladder can comfortably hold through the night, either your kidneys produce an abnormally large volume of urine at night or your bladder capacity is reduced. Of course, it is also possible to have both conditions. Making too much urine overnight is called nocturnal polyuria (polyuria means excessive urine output). Common causes of nocturnal polyuria and reduced bladder capacity are listed in Table 1.

The key to diagnosing the cause of nocturia is the voiding diary. To keep a voiding diary, you record the time and amount (using a measuring cup) of each urination for a 24- to 48-hour period. The total volume that you urinate for a 24-hour period is calculated. Urinating more than about 2.5 liters during the day is considered to be polyuria. If you void a normal amount over 24 hours, but greater than one-third of your total volume of urine is produced overnight, that is considered to be nocturnal polyuria. Next, you compare the largest volume that you urinate during the day to the largest overnight volume. If you wake up at night to urinate, but the largest overnight volume is less than the largest volume of urine voided during the day, the problem is reduced overnight bladder capacity, called nocturnal detrusor overactivity. Let's look at some examples.

61

Table 1. Common Causes of Nocturia

A. Nocturnal polyuria
   1. Cardiac (heart) failure
   2. Peripheral edema (swollen legs)
   3. Excessive fluid intake (polydipsia)
      a. Diabetes mellitus
      b. Diabetes insipidus
      c. Habit
      d. Psychogenic
      e. Iatrogenic
         1. Lithium toxicity
         2. Anticholinergics
   4. Diuretics
B. Reduced bladder capacity
   1. Bladder or prostate infection
   2. Benign prostatic hyperplasia
      (enlarged prostate)
   3. Bladder or prostate cancer
   4. Interstitial cystitis
   5. Detrusor overactivity
      a. Neurogenic bladder
      b. Detrusor instability

Polly is a 41-year-old married woman, the personnel director of a large department store. Until recently, she led a very active life and was an avid tennis player, but for the last several months has been plagued by having to get up three to five times every night to urinate. She has difficulty falling back to sleep and is tired all the time. She no longer engages in any of the things she loves to do. She said that she voids about every two hours during the day and denied any other symptoms at all. She had a normal physical examination and urinalysis. Her voiding diary is shown in Figure 1.

Polly went to sleep at midnight and was awakened three times to urinate before finally arising at 7:15 AM for the day. She voided 1600 ml during sleeping hours (1600 ml/5035 ml = 32%). The upper limit for normal overnight urine output is 35% of the 24-hour output, so she does not have nocturnal polyuria. You can see that Polly has a 24-hour urinary output of over 5 liters. That is more than twice the upper limit of normal, and more than three times what an average person urinates. Her nighttime voided volumes are more than double her average daytime volume, and as noted, her total volume overnight is less than a third of her 24-hour volume. Her bladder holds plenty; Polly's only problem is that she makes too much urine. Why does Polly make so much urine. It's simple; she drinks too

NAME: Polly

Time of void	Voided volume (ml)	Incontinence (S, U, W) see below	Amount of leakage (Large = L, Medium = M, Small = S)
7:00 AM	200		
7:45	125		
8:50	150		
10:30	225		
11:00	150		
11:20	100		
12:55 PM	100		
1:30	200		
1:50	110		
2:30	250		
4:00	375		
5:30	275		
6:15	150		
8:00	225		
9:00	350		
9:20	200		
11:00	250		
12:30 AM	400		
1:30	450		
4:30	550		
7:15	200		
Total	5035		

Incontinence is the loss of urine control before reaching the bathroom.

S = Stress incontinence is wetting or leakage at times of coughing, sneezing, or with physical activity, etc.

U = Urge incontinence is wetting or leakage because of urgency.

W = Unaware incontinence is wetting without conscious awareness of when it happens.

Figure 1. Polly's voiding diary.

much water. She carries a plastic water bottle during the day because she thinks it's healthy to drink a lot of water to cleanse her system. For most people, it's OK to do that, but if you drink that much fluid during the day, you'll make a lot of urine and, like Polly, you'll probably be up at night to urinate. Polly threw away her water bottle and she's sleeping through the night, playing tennis, and doing all the other things she missed.

Mrs. Nusog is a 72-year-old manic-depressive, but you'd never know it. She is a well-respected artistic director for a theater company and her psychiatric condition has been nearly perfectly controlled for over 30 years with lithium. Her voiding diary looked just like Polly's. I told her to stop drinking so much water, but she told me that she wasn't drinking much at all; she said that she only drinks because she is thirsty. She did another diary and this time recorded how much she ate and drank. She drank over 3.5 liters in a single day, more than three times normal. We went over the diary and she agreed to get on a schedule, cutting back on her fluids by 50%. When she came back one week later, she still drank about 3.5 liters a day, still voided over 5 liters, and she still got up at night to urinate. Mrs. Nusog simply couldn't stop drinking; she became too thirsty. After a series of blood and urine tests, it was discovered that her excessive thirst was due to the lithium that she had been taking for so long. Under the care of her psychiatrist, the lithium was discontinued and she was started on another medication. It took a long time, nearly four months, but her condition finally reversed itself and she's nearly back to normal.

Overall, polyuria is not that common a cause of nocturia; in my experience it accounts for about 10% of nocturia cases, but if that's what's causing your symptoms, and they are not caused by a more serious condition like diabetes mellitus or diabetes insipidus, the treatment is usually fairly straightforward. Just stop drinking so much. If you can't stop drinking, it is very important that you undergo a careful diagnostic evaluation to rule out the more serious causes.

Many patients complain mainly of nocturia, but when questioned, it turns out that they have many more symptoms than that. Older men, for example, when questioned may complain of daytime frequency, urgency, and weak stream, but what bothers them the most is nocturia because it interferes with their sleep. Consider the case of Harry, a retired waiter who complained that he was getting up every hour and a half at night to urinate. He also voided every hour during the day and had urgency several times a day. The daytime symptoms, although quite severe, didn't bother him at all because he was always near a bathroom. What really bothered him was getting up at night so often. His voiding diary is depicted in Figure 2.

NAME: Harry
PLEASE RECORD THIS DIARY FOR ONE 24-HOUR PERIOD.
PLEASE READ VOIDING DIARY INSTRUCTIONS.
Instructions: Place an "X" in the spaces provided if any of these symptoms occur while urinating or trying to urinate.

Time of void	Amount in ml	Urgency	Push or strain	Incomplete voiding	Start and stop	Weak stream
6:30 AM	240	X	X		X	X
7:15	60	X				X
8:30	30	X				X
9:10	30	X		X		X
11:15	90					X
1:15 PM	90					X
3:30	60			X		X
5:50	60	X	X	X		X
7:45	30					X
10:00	90					X
11:50	30	X				X
12:30 AM	150					X
1:05	190	X				X
2:30	240					X
3:15	200	X		X	X	X
4:00	200					
5:15	150					
6:30	240	X	X	X		X
Total	2180					

Figure 2. Harry's voiding diary.

The diary shows that he voided over 2 liters in 24 hours, but that nearly 1.4 liters was made during his sleep from 11:50 PM until 6:30 AM (1400 ml/2180 ml = 64%). Thus, he has nocturnal polyuria. Further, the largest volume he ever voided during the day was only 90 ml; that's only 3 oz! At night, though, he voided over twice that amount each time he urinated. Harry has two problems. He has an enlarged prostate, which causes a blockage to the flow of urine, and his legs swell a bit toward the end of the day. The swelling in his legs, an accumulation of fluid called *edema*, is caused by a condition called venous insufficiency. When he lies down at night to go to sleep, the fluid in his legs is absorbed into his bloodstream and filtered by his kidneys, so Harry makes a lot more urine during the night (when he is lying down) than during the day (when he is standing all the time).

Even though his symptoms were severe, all Harry wanted was to be able to sleep at night. He would probably have benefited tremendously from prostate surgery, but he didn't even want to consider it. Harry was told to wear elastic stockings during the day to keep the swelling in his legs down and he was also treated with doxazocin (Cardura). Doxazocin is an alpha blocker, a medication that relaxes the muscles in the wall of the prostate and helps to relieve the blockage to the flow of urine. On this regimen, Harry's edema was very mild and he got up only once a night to urinate. An added benefit was that his daytime frequency was dramatically reduced and he found urination to be much easier.

Venous insufficiency like Harry's is very common. Another common condition that causes exactly the same problem is mild heart failure. You would think that if you had heart failure either *you or your doctor* would know about it, but that's often not the case. Sometimes the only symptom of heart failure is nocturia. When heart failure is the cause, it is usually quite treatable.

Minnie, an 88-year-old widow, had almost identical complaints as Harry, but Minnie doesn't have a prostate and her legs don't swell either. Take a look at Minnie's diary (Figure 3).

Minnie voided less than 1 liter in 24 hours, yet she urinated more than half of that overnight, so she had nocturnal polyuria. The largest amount that she ever urinated at one time was only 120 ml; Minnie had a very small bladder capacity. She underwent a complete medical and urologic evaluation, but no cause for either problem was discovered. Minnie was started on a medication called desmopression (DDAVP) at bedtime. DDAVP is a medicine that temporarily reduces the amount of urine that the kidneys produce. She was cured of her nocturia, but during the day, when the kidneys made up for the urine not produced at night, she began to urinate even more frequently. She then underwent a three-month course of behavior modification. During that time, she met with a behavioral therapist once a week and gradually learned to increase the time between urinations until her bladder could comfortably hold over 300 ml. Now she urinates about every three hours and gets up only once at night to urinate.

NAME: Minnie
PLEASE RECORD THIS DIARY FOR ONE 24-HOUR PERIOD.
PLEASE READ VOIDING DIARY INSTRUCTIONS.
Instructions: Place an "X" in the spaces provided if any of these symptoms occur while urinating or trying to urinate.

Time of void	Amount in ml	Urgency	Push or strain	Incomplete voiding	Start and stop	Weak stream
6:15 AM	100	X				
8:45	30	X				X
10:00	30	X				X
11:15	30	X		X		X
12:15 PM	30					X
2:45	45					X
3:30	30			X		X
5:15	30	X				X
7:50	45					X
10:00	30					X
12:30 AM	90	X				
1:40	90	X				
2:55	120	X				
4:30	120	X				
6:00	120	X		X	X	
Total	940					

Figure 3. Minnie's voiding diary.

Another elderly woman had the same symptoms as Minnie, but her urinalysis showed microscopic hematuria (traces of blood in the urine that are not visible to the naked eye). After evaluation, including cystoscopy, she was found to have bladder cancer. She underwent a minor surgical procedure called transurethral resection for the bladder tumor and, so far, she's OK.

As you can see, each of these people had fairly similar symptoms, but the causes were very different. Sometimes, the problem is nothing more than drinking too much fluid; other times, it's a serious condition like bladder or prostate cancer. For that reason, even if the symptoms don't bother you, it's important that you see a doctor.

WHAT SHOULD THE DOCTOR DO?

The first thing the doctor should do is always the same: take a detailed history about your complaints, then do a physical examination. Some causes of nocturia are obvious on history and examination. For example, on history and examination of your heart and lungs, congestive heart failure can be readily diagnosed. By examination of your legs, particularly late in the day, edema and signs of venous insufficiency can be detected. A urinalysis should be done. If there is blood in the urine, whether visible to the naked eye or not, that should be fully evaluated. If a bladder infection is diagnosed, it should be treated with antibiotics. If no obvious cause is found, your doctor should ask you to complete a voiding diary. Based on the diary, the cause of your nocturia should be categorized as either nocturnal polyuria, a small-capacity bladder, or a combination of both conditions. Further evaluation depends on the specifics of your condition, but no matter what the cause, after proper evaluation, there is almost always a successful way to treat nocturia.

Nevertheless, certain generalities about the evaluation should be mentioned. If the problem is small bladder capacity, and neither infection nor hematuria is found, the next step is urodynamic evaluation (see Chapter 4). Urodynamics refers to one or more tests of a series that are designed to diagnose the cause of your bladder symptoms. A small catheter is passed through your urethra into the bladder. Usually another catheter is passed into the rectum. The bladder is filled with fluid to simulate natural filling of urine from the kidneys. During bladder filling, you will be asked about your sensations and you'll be checked for incontinence. When you get the urge, you'll be asked to urinate. During this whole process, the pressure in the bladder and rectum are monitored and, in most instances, the exact cause of your symptoms can be determined. After the urodynamic evaluation, depending on the results, you may need to undergo cystoscopy (looking into the bladder) as well.

If nocturnal polyuria is the problem, or part of the problem, a thorough medical evaluation by your doctor, including a battery of blood tests, will probably be necessary.

TREATMENT OF NOCTURIA

Treatment is dependent on the underlying cause. For remediable conditions such as urinary tract infection, congestive heart failure, diabetes mellitus, diabetes insipdus, and so forth, treatment of the underlying condition usually cures the nocturia. In many patients, though, the cause is not so obvious, and empiric therapy must be tried. For people with nocturnal polyuria, treatment is directed at decreasing the amount of urine that the kidneys produce overnight. There are three ways of accomplishing this—by fluid restriction, by the use of diuretics, and by the use of DDAVP. A fairly simple way of beginning is to decrease the amount of food and fluid that you ingest at dinner and in the evening hours. Many people, particularly elderly men and women, drink a lot more than they need to in the evening. Not infrequently, they've been told by doctors or friends that it's important to drink eight glasses of water a day; others drink a lot of fluid because they take a lot of pills. No matter what the reason though, if you drink a lot at dinner or in the evening, the chances are that you'll get up a lot at night to urinate.

Another way of decreasing nighttime urinary volume is by taking DDAVP just before you go to bed at night, like Minnie. Remember though, it works by slowing down the production of urine for eight hours or so. When you wake up, your kidneys will begin to make all the urine that they should have made overnight and you'll have to urinate more during the day or learn to hold a larger amount in your bladder. Finally, there are diuretics. These are medications that cause the kidneys to make more urine.

I don't understand. Why would I take a medication that causes my kidneys to make more urine?

The idea is to take the diuretic during the day, usually in the late afternoon, so that you get rid of all the excess fluid in your body before you got to sleep for the night.

All three of these methods can be very effective, but in the beginning they may require a lot of effort on your part and on your doctor's part. You've got to experiment not only with the right dose, but also with the timing of when you take the medications or withhold your fluids so that you can get a good night's sleep. It will probably require a fair amount of record keeping and diaries before you get it just right, but if you persist, the treatment will probably work.

For empirical treatment of small-capacity bladder, I believe that behavior modification should be tried first. It worked for Minnie and it will probably work for you, but it's work; it's not a pill. You'll have to see a behavioral therapist once a week or so and you'll have to keep diaries and records. The treatments can be time consuming and expensive, but it can work. When it does work, it's a cure and there are no possible complications. To do it properly requires motivation, so if you're not motivated or don't believe in it, it's probably not going to work. With the proper therapist, it's really all up to you.

Some people are unwilling to do behavior modification because they don't believe in it or they think it's too much trouble. I think that's a mistake, but it's your decision. If you have a small-capacity bladder and you're unwilling to try behavior modification, there are some medications that can be used empirically—DDAVP, diuretics, anticholinergics, and tricyclic antidepressants. You already know about DDAVP and diuretics. Anticholinergics such as oxybutynin (Ditropan) and tricyclic antidepressants like imipramine (Tofranil) are intended to work by stopping the bladder from contracting involuntarily. If that's what's making you get up at night they may work, but I'd still vote for behavior modification because it works for involuntary bladder contractions too.

CONCLUSION

Nocturia, or getting up to urinate after you go to sleep at night is one of the most common and one of the most bothersome of symptoms. The key to diagnosis is a thorough medical evaluation including urinalysis and a voiding diary. It is important to undergo a thorough evaluation because sometimes the symptoms are caused by a serious condition like heart failure or bladder cancer. On the basis of the evaluation, the cause of nocturia can be classified as either excessive overnight production of urine (nocturnal polyuria), small-capacity bladder, or a combination of the two. Fortunately, when treatment is based on knowledge of the underlying cause, it is almost always treatable and curable.

7

Bedwetting

INTRODUCTION

If you look up the word enuresis in the dictionary, you'll find that it means involuntary urination. Nocturnal enuresis, commonly known as bedwetting, simply means urinary incontinence that occurs at night, when you are sleeping. However, in medical circles, enuresis is used as a synonym for bedwetting, not as a synonym for incontinence. Of course, if you work at night and sleep during the day, and you wet your bed when you're sleeping, it's the same problem. It's bedwetting, but it's not nocturnal enuresis. When you think of enuresis, you undoubtedly think of children and toilet training, but adults can have enuresis too. Enuresis can be categorized into two general types, primary and secondary enuresis. Primary enuresis means that the person was never successfully toilet trained and wet the bed for as long as he or she can remember. In secondary enuresis, the person was successfully toilet trained and confidently dry at night for a period of time, but subsequently developed bedwetting.

ENURESIS IN CHILDREN

Normally, children begin to gain some daytime continence by about $1\frac{1}{2}$–2 years of age, but it is rare for a child to achieve nighttime continence before that age. After $1\frac{1}{2}$ years of age, about 20% of children gain continence per year until about age $4\frac{1}{2}$, and a smaller amount gain continence each year thereafter until, by age 10, 95% of children have nearly perfect day and night control. By puberty, only 2% of children still have any problems with incontinence. Learning to control urination is part of maturation, yet it is a very complex neurophysiological and behavioral process. At birth, voiding is a simple reflex—the bladder fills with urine from the kidneys and when a certain threshold is reached the sphincter relaxes, the bladder contracts, and voiding occurs. This is called the micturition reflex. As the child grows and the neurologic system begins to mature, he or she begins to develop a sense of urge to urinate, and eventually (hopefully) learns that some times and places are better than others for voiding. With further maturation, he or she eventually learns how to contract the sphincter and prevent or abort the bladder contraction, and finally, the child learns how to delay micturition for longer and longer periods of time until complete day and night continence is achieved. Finally, the child learns to initiate urination voluntarily, even before the bladder is completely full. Experts pretty much agree that by age $2\frac{1}{2}$–3 years, the components of the nervous system that are involved with voluntary control of micturition have sufficiently matured, but the cognitive and learning skills that are necessary are not fully operable until about $4\frac{1}{2}$ years of age.

As you all know, along the way to achieving bladder control, there are many mishaps. Some are made by the children themselves, even more are probably made by overzealous parents who embark on toilet training before the child is ready. Since the age at which children become fully continent is so variable, it's not possible to pick a specific age at which to be concerned if a child is not yet toilet trained. A good general rule of thumb, though, is that you should be concerned when it is of psychosocial concern to your child. Of course, *your concerns* are of psychosocial concern to your child, so if you make a big deal out of it, so will your child. If you make a big deal out of it before your child's nervous system has matured to the point where he or she can be toilet trained, that's an even bigger deal! Nevertheless for most children, it becomes an important concern between about ages 5 and 7 years.

Causes of Enuresis in Children

Theoretically, the causes of enuresis in children are the same as the causes of urinary incontinence at any age, but children are overwhelmingly more likely to have an overactive bladder rather than a weak sphincter. The likely causes of childhood enuresis are listed in Table 1. In most children, bedwetting occurs because the bladder contracts involuntarily and incontinence ensues when the child fails to wake up in time to stop it. The reasons why the bladder might contract involuntarily at night are exactly the same as the reasons why it would contract involuntarily during the day, and, in fact, many children with enuresis took longer to

Table 1. Causes of Bedwetting in Children

Because of the bladder:
1. Involuntary detrusor contractions
    A. Detrusor instability
        1. Idiopathic
        2. Urinary tract infection
        3. Posterior urethral valves
    B. Detrusor hyperreflexia
        1. Maturation defect
        2. Spina bifida (myelodysplasia)
        3. Spinal cord tumor
2. Lower bladder compliance
    A. Neurogenic
        1. Spina bifida (myelodysplasia)
        2. Spinal cord tumor
Because of the sphincter:
1. Intrinsic sphincter deficiency
    A. Neurogenic
        1. Spina bifida (myelodysplasia)
        2. Spinal cord tumor
    B. Postsurgical

achieve daytime continence in the first place. Most episodes of enuresis occur during non–rapid eye movement sleep, a time of very deep sleep. For this reason, for many years it was believed that deep sleep is the main cause of enuresis. However, many subsequent studies have shown that enuretic children do not sleep any deeper than nonenuretic children and that deep sleepers are no more likely to be enuretic than normal sleepers. Thus, deep sleep itself is not the primary cause of enuresis, although it is certainly possible that it contributes to the problem.

Another theory about the cause of bedwetting is that children make more urine at night than normal. This is thought to be caused by a reversal of the normal circadian rhythm of antidiuretic hormone secretion. In simple terms, this means that some children make more urine during sleeping hours than during the day because of an abnormality in the secretion of an antidiuretic hormone (ADH, or vasopressin) that regulates urine production. Normally, a child makes more urine during the day than during the night. The overnight production of urine is less than the bladder can comfortably hold, so he or she doesn't have to wake up at night to urinate and there is no reason for the bladder to contract involuntarily. The reason that less urine is made overnight is because there is an increased production of ADH at night. ADH, a substance produced by the pituitary gland in the brain, signals the kidneys to cut back on urine production. ADH is normally secreted in a rhythmic fashion, reaching its peak at about the same time each night. This cyclic production of ADH is called a circadian rhythm.

Research has shown that many enuretic children (and maybe some adults) have a reversal of the normal circadian rhythm of ADH production, so they make more urine at night than their bladder can comfortably hold. Of course, simply making more urine at night is not the only factor in enuresis because, once toilet training has been achieved, the normal child has learned to inhibit the micturition reflex whenever he or she wants to. If there is enuresis, it must mean that the child is sleeping so deeply that he or she never feels a thing and just urinates during sleep.

For the great majority of children with enuresis, the cause is never determined and eventually the child outgrows it; remember, by puberty, no more than 2% of children still have enuresis. Some researchers believe that environmental factors also play an important role. For example, there is an increased incidence of enuresis in children from broken homes and from lower socioeconomic classes. On the other hand, genetic factors cannot be ignored because there is an increased incidence of enuresis in twins who were the result of fertilization of a single egg (monozygotic twins) compared to dizygotic twins, who come from two different eggs. Monozygotic twins share exactly the same genetic makeup, whereas dizygotic twins have different genes from both mother and father. Further, enuresis tends to run in families, and when it does, continence is generally achieved at about the same age from generation to generation. For example, if a person was not fully toilet trained until age 7, the chances are that his or her child won't be toilet trained until the same age.

In childhood, enuresis is divided into primary and secondary enuresis. In primary enuresis, the child has never achieved complete continence for more than a few days at a time; in secondary enuresis complete day and night continence had been achieved for a prolonged period of time before the incontinence occurred. Of note, about 85% of children with nocturnal enuresis have daytime incontinence as well. Further, about 10–25% of children with enuresis are still not fully continent of stool. Incontinence of stool is called encopresis. Most enuretic children are boys (male:female ratio is 3:2).

Evaluation of Enuresis in Children

There are many crucial aspects to the evaluation of enuresis in childhood. If not diagnosed and treated appropriately and if not handled with love, care, and understanding, the consequences of enuresis can leave severe emotional and psychological scars that can last a lifetime. Further, even though they are uncommon, some causes of enuresis can be life threatening and/or have severe medical consequences.

The evaluation begins with a detailed account of the type and onset of symptoms. It is important that the child be an integral part of the history taking and that he or she participate in the evaluation process. A physical exam by his or her doctor should be done to be sure that there are no obvious causes of enuresis such as a distended bladder or neurologic abnormalities. Often, the neurologic abnormalities may be very subtle; for example, a dimple or discoloration on the back, just above the buttock crease, especially if there is a patch of hair there, may signal the presence of a previously undiagnosed spina bifida. A high arching of the feet or atrophy of the small muscles of the feet also suggest spina bifida. Incontinence associated with a sudden growth spurt suggests the possibility of a tethered spinal cord. A tethered spinal cord is one that is scarred to the bony spinal canal, most often seen in children with spina bifida. It may cause no symptoms until the child starts to grow. Then, the bones of the spine grow faster than the nerves. The nerves become stretched and damaged and eventually can cause symptoms including incontinence. Other symptoms relate to the muscles that are innervated by the stretched nerves.

A urinalysis should be done to exclude urinary tract infection, which is probably the most common cause of secondary enuresis. Often, even when there is a urinary tract infection, there are no other symptoms except for enuresis. If infection is found, the symptoms generally subside after treatment with an antibiotic, but if they persist or recur, a careful search for the cause of infections should be made. Of particular importance in this regard is to be sure that infections are not being caused by congenital anatomic abnormalities such as vesicoureteral reflux or posterior urethral valves.

What's vesicoureteral reflux? What's posterior urethral valves?

These are the two most common known remedial causes of urinary tract infections in children. Although neither of these conditions actually causes urinary tract infection, once bacteria have entered the bladder, for whatever reason, the bacteria and the infection are much more difficult to clear. Further, these two conditions probably lower the defense mechanisms against infections in the first place. *Vesicoureteral reflux* means that there is a backflow of urine from the bladder to the kidneys. Normally, the kidneys make urine that is transported to the bladder through the two thin muscular tubes called ureters (see Chapter 2). Once it enters the bladder, urine is prevented from backing (refluxing) into the ureters because of the way in which the ureters enter the bladder and some other muscular properties of the bladder and ureter themselves. Thus, it is said that the ureters are normally nonrefluxing. Vesicoureteral reflux occurs if there is an abnormality in the course of the ureter as it enters the bladder or if the pressure in the bladder gets too high. High pressure in the bladder may be caused by low bladder compliance, mostly from neurologic conditions such as spina bifida, or from a blockage to urine flow through the urethra. In boys, such a blockage is almost always caused by posterior urethral valves. In girls, a blockage is almost unheard of.

Posterior urethral valves is a congenital abnormality that, for practical purposes, only affects boys. The valves are really birth defects, little leaflets or flaps of tissue in the urethra of boys that can cause very severe obstruction. Like most things, there is a wide spectrum of clinical presentation of posterior urethral valves. Some cause only mild obstruction with few symptoms that the boy outgrows in time; others are so severe that the baby is stillborn or dies shortly after birth. In the more severe cases, boys who survive the neonatal period usually present with recurrent urinary tract infections, most often with high fever that is unexplained until urinalysis is done. Other boys present only with enuresis.

Now, let's return to the diagnostic evaluation. If the urinalysis shows infection or blood in the urine, that needs to be evaluated to determine the cause. If not, the next step is to have the child do a diary and pad test. The diary simply records the time and amount of each urination and whether or not the child had any conscious awareness of the actual moment of urinary loss, whether during the day or night. Based on the diary and the child's own account of symptoms, there are several possibilities. It may be apparent that his or her bladder simply doesn't hold enough, day or night. For example, if the largest urination event during the day is only 150 ml (5 oz.) and the child makes 300 ml (10 oz.) of urine overnight, it is obvious that something has to give. Either he or she has to wake up at night to urinate (nocturia) or, if the child is a deep sleeper, the bed will be wet. If the child makes 500 ml (17 oz.) all day and 900 (30 oz.) all night, the problem is a reversal of the normal circadian ADH cycle. Of course, it is possible (and common) for both of these problems to exist concomitantly.

Treatment of Childhood Enuresis

Treatment, of course, should be predicated on a clear understanding of the physiological abnormalities causing the condition—infection, small bladder capacity, involuntary bladder contractions, reversal of the circadian ADH cycle, etc. If infection is found, it should be treated and if it doesn't recur, there is no need for further evaluation in a girl. In a boy, because infections usually have an underlying congenital/anatomic cause, a full urologic evaluation should be done.

If there is no infection, treatment will depend very much on the results of the diary and pad test. Punishment, harsh words, a disapproving glance, reprimand, and derisive remarks are absolutely taboo. They serve no useful purpose and only serve to lower the child's self-esteem and generally result in regressive behavior. For most children, I believe the best course of treatment is behavior modification. Merely having the child fill out the diary form immediately involves the child in the treatment program. If that is supplemented by a positive and hopeful attitude on the part of therapists, parents, and siblings, a successful outcome is nearly guaranteed. When bladder capacity is small, behavior modification is directed at a purposeful and gradual increase in bladder capacity. This is done by having the child keep a voiding diary, and based on that diary, a schedule for the following week is planned. In general, it is best to try to increase the time between urinations by about 15 minutes per week until the child can comfortably hold more urine during the day than his or her overnight production of urine.

If overnight production of urine is excessive, first look to be sure that the child is not drinking or eating an excessive amount in the late afternoon or evening. If not, an empirical trial with a synthetic analogue of ADH, called DDAVP, is the next step. DDAVP acts in just the same way as ADH. It decreases the production of urine by the kidneys. It is generally given in the form of a nasal spray just before bedtime. One or two sprays is generally all that is needed. Each spray contains 10 μg of DDAVP, so 10–20 μg is the usual dose. DDAVP has proven to be very safe; I am not aware of any serious complications in children. However, it is a potentially dangerous drug if it is not administered properly. Each spray is a dose, like a pill. One spray is 10 μg, two sprays is 20 μg, 3 sprays 30 μg, and so on. If a child takes too much of the medication, the kidneys would not make any urine for a long time and, if he or she continued to drink, overhydration could occur. This could result in dilution of the normal chemicals in the blood and could cause seizures, high blood pressure, and even heart failure. As I mentioned, this has never been reported in children, but you must be aware of it and not give more than your doctor prescribes. And, certainly, don't give more in the daytime because it worked so well at night.

Other behavioral approaches are also used. One of the more popular is the bell-and-alarm system. The child is hooked up to an electronic alarm system that senses the first drop of urine as it comes out at night. Two electrodes are placed on the child's underwear or bed. When urine touches them, it completes an electronic circuit, which makes a bell or vibrator go off, waking up the child. Although it doesn't prevent that episode of incontinence, it does two things. First, it documents when the incontinence occurs so that the child can be awakened beforehand the next night and asked to urinate to prevent the incontinence. Second, it serves to heighten the child's awareness and he or she might subconsciously learn to abort the involuntary detrusor contraction that led to the enuresis in the first place.

Even though I think that behavioral approaches are best, most doctors use medications. The most popular medication is imipramine (Tofranil). It is a time-honored approach and reportedly successful in about 40% of children. Imipramine, as I mentioned in Chapter 5, is a tricyclic antidepressant that has very specific effects on the bladder, reducing the frequency of involuntary bladder contractions. In children, the usual dose is about 1–1.5 mg/kg/day (2–3 mg/lb/day) given at bedtime or in the late afternoon, depending on when the child usually wets the bed. Anticholinergic medications such as oxybutynin (Ditropan), propantheline (ProBanthine) and hyoscyamine (Levsin) are also sometimes used.

ENURESIS IN ADULTS

As you've just seen, in children, enuresis is almost always a problem of maturation that, even if untreated, resolves itself in time. Not so in adults, particularly adult men. The onset of enuresis in adults is most often the result of a more serious underlying problem. This means that if a man or woman develops enuresis, it demands prompt evaluation and treatment.

Causes of Enuresis in Adults

In adult men with secondary enuresis, severe prostatic or vesical neck obstruction is by far the most common cause; in women, it's probably a previously undiagnosed neurologic condition. After urethral obstruction, neurologic conditions are the second most common cause in men. Neurologic conditions can cause enuresis by one of two mechanisms. First, the bladder may cease to work at all, leaving a large amount of residual urine in the bladder that simply spills over at night; this is called overflow incontinence. Overflow incontinence is most commonly seen with ruptured discs, spinal cord tumors, and spina bifida. It is also seen after operations for cancer of the female cervix and uterus and in both sexes after surgery for rectal cancer. Second, there may be involuntary bladder contractions that result in incontinence. This is most often seen with such conditions as multiple sclerosis, cerebrovascular accident, Parkinson's disease, and other degenerative neurologic diseases. A more complete list of the most common causes of enuresis in adults is seen in Table 2.

Table 2. Causes of Bedwetting in Adults

Because of the bladder:
1. Involuntary bladder contractions
    A. Detrusor instability (involuntary bladder contractions in the absence of an underlying neurologic condition)
        1. Prostatic urethral obstruction (in men)
        2. Bladder neck obstruction (mostly men, some women)
        3. Bladder or prostate infection
    B. Detrusor hyperreflexia (involuntary bladder contractions due to an underlying neurologic condition)
        1. Multiple sclerosis
        2. CVA
        3. Brain tumor
        4. Transverse myelitis
        5. Spina bifida (myelodysplasia)
        6. Spinal cord tumor
2. Low bladder compliance
    A. Neurogenic
        1. Transverse myelitis
        2. Spina bifida (myelodysplasia)
        3. Spinal cord tumor
    B. Nonneurogenic
        1. Prostatic urethral obstruction
        2. Radiation cystitis
        3. Tuberculous cystitis
3. Weak or absent bladder contractions
    A. Nonneurogenic (idiopathic)
    B. Neurogenic
        1. Occult spina bifida (myelodysplasia)
        2. Spinal cord tumor
        3. Transverse myelitis
        4. Ruptured disc
Because of the sphincter:
1. Nonneurogenic
    A. Intrinsic sphincter deficiency in women
    B. After prostate surgery in men
2. Neurogenic
    A. Spina bifida (myelodysplasia)
    B. Spinal cord tumor
    C. Transverse myelitis
    D. Ruptured disc

Do you mean that if a man or woman develops bedwetting at night, without any other symptoms at all, there could be a serious underlying cause?

That's exactly what I mean. Of course it is possible to have an occasional episode of enuresis if you've had too much alcohol to drink and you pass out in your bed, but hopefully that doesn't happen very often. Further, if you already have incontinence during the day, then nighttime incontinence is most likely caused by the same condition. However, if you develop recurrent enuresis, even without any other symptoms at all, you should have a thorough evaluation by a urologist. Let me give you a couple of examples:

Stanley is a healthy stockbroker, married with two children, whose only symptom was that he started urinating a little more frequently than usual, about every two hours during the day. He attributed this to the fact that he drank about 10 cups of coffee a day while at work. For several weeks he had been wetting the bed during the night without waking up. He saw his family doctor, who obtained a urinalysis, which was normal. He was referred to a urologist who examined him and measured his postvoid residual urine with an ultrasound. To the astonishment of both patient and doctor, Stanley had a residual urine of over 1500 ml; that's over 1 gallon! And that is after he had already urinated 600 ml, so he actually held over 2 gallons in his bladder and didn't even know it. Blood tests showed that he was in renal failure (his serum creatinine was 2.5) and renal ultrasound showed that both kidneys were obstructed—he had bilateral hydronephrosis. *Hydronephrosis* means that there has been damage to the kidney because of a blockage. Video-urodynamic study showed severe obstruction by the prostate, and fortunately, after prostatic surgery (transurethral resection of the prostate), his kidneys returned to normal and the enuresis subsided. Further, he now voids in normal amounts and has only a small amount of residual urine.

Stanley was lucky. The enuresis, which in itself was not so terrible a symptom, was a warning sign of a potentially fatal condition that was completely reversed by surgery.

Eric, a movie producer, was not quite so fortunate. He also developed enuresis and had no other symptoms at all. On evaluation, he was also found to have an enormous bladder; it held over 2 liters. But in Eric's case the cause was a spinal cord tumor called an ependymoma. As he was being evaluated, before the eyes of his doctors, he became paraplegic, unable to move his legs at all. After spinal surgery to remove the tumor, he was eventually able to walk again, but his bladder never recovered and he now must do intermittent self-catheterization four times a day in place of urinating. Aside from that, though, he is doing very well. He works full time, he still produces movies, and, by his own account, "life is pretty good."

I don't understand. These are all serious diseases. Why do they only cause symptoms at night?

Most of the time they do cause symptoms day and night, but sometimes, particularly in the early stages, they may present only with enuresis. The likely explanation is that during the day there is a heightened sense of awareness compared to during sleep. People with these problems may subconsciously begin to urinate more frequently or drink less fluid to prevent daytime incontinence.

Evaluation of Adults with Enuresis

As always, the evaluation begins by your doctor asking a bunch of questions: When did it start? Are there any other symptoms? Are there symptoms of urinary tract infection such as pain during urination or marked frequency? Are there signs of a blockage in the urethra such as weak stream or difficulty starting? Are there signs of a neurologic condition like numbness or tingling or weakness in the arms or legs? On the initial visit, a urinalysis and urine culture should be done to make sure that the enuresis is not being caused by a simple infection. If infection is found, it should be treated with culture-specific antibiotics and, in the majority of women, that's all that needs to be done. In men, infections are much less common than in women and are usually caused by an underlying condition such as prostatic obstruction. For this reason, even if infection is found to be the cause, after you've been treated, it is important to have a urologic evaluation. In either sex, if there is blood in the urine, a full workup including a kidney X ray and cystoscopy (looking into the bladder) should be done.

The next step in evaluation is for you to get a uroflow and postvoid residual urine determination. For the uroflow, you simply urinate into a funnel that measures the urinary flow rate and the amount of urine that you voided. The amount of urine that is left in your bladder after urinating, the postvoid residual (PVR), is usually measured with an ultrasound probe placed over your lower abdomen immediately after you urinate. Both the uroflow and PVR determinations are noninvasive and painless and they give very important information. If the residual urine is high and the flow is low and you are a man, the chances are that you have a blockage in the urethra, most likely from the prostate. If you are a woman, you most likely have a weak bladder. If you've had previous pelvic surgery, there may be a blockage due to scarring in the urethra. No matter what the results of the uroflow and residual—even if they are normal—the next step is urodynamics. In either case, the only means of making an accurate diagnosis is to perform urodynamic studies as outlined in Chapter 4. If a urethral obstruction is found, the specific cause should be investigated. This will probably require cystoscopy to see exactly where in the urethra the blockage is. If the bladder is found to be weakened or not working at all, or if there are unexplained involuntary bladder contractions, it may be necessary to see a neurologist to evaluate the possibility of a neurologic condition like Eric had.

Treatment of Adult Enuresis

Treatment should be predicated on a clear understanding of the underlying cause. Of course, if the enuresis is a symptom of a neurologic condition like multiple sclerosis or spinal cord tumor, those conditions must be fully evaluated and treated whenever possible. In some situations, treatment of the neurologic condition will cure the enuresis; in other cases, like Eric's, a specific treatment will need to be tailored to the individual.

In men, the most common cause of enuresis is a urethral blockage by the prostate or bladder neck. Treatment may be begun with alpha-adrenergic blocking agents such as terazocin (Hytrin) or doxazocin (Cardura), but these are only effective in a minority of men. More likely, prostatic or bladder neck surgery will be necessary. If you want to find out more about these things, see Chapter 12. If overflow incontinence is the cause, it is still possible (and likely) that the underlying problem is urethral obstruction, which should be treated as just discussed. If the bladder doesn't work at all, a careful search for a neurologic etiology should be undertaken, but in the meantime, intermittent self-catheterization should be begun. Self intermittent catheterization (SIC) is a means of emptying the bladder when you cannot urinate normally. It may be used as a temporary method while you are awaiting or undergoing treatment, or it may be part of a permanent treatment program. With this technique, you pass a catheter through the urethra into your bladder to empty the urine. It is usually done three to six times a day, depending on how much urine your bladder can safely hold. Even though it sounds gruesome, SIC is actually quite safe, easy, and painless. Only in the rarest of circumstances should an indwelling catheter be used. This may be necessary if the person is unable to catheterize himself or herself because of severe disability.

Even women can have overflow incontinence and enuresis as the result of a urethral obstruction, but it is exceedingly rare unless the woman has had prior urethral surgery. Consider the case of Suzanne, a 53-year-old, married art dealer. For as long as she could remember she had urinated much less frequently than her friends; she could go all day without voiding even once! Then she had a single episode of enuresis and she happened to mention it to her gynecologist, who, on examination, felt an enormous pelvic mass. He thought she had ovarian cancer, but ultrasound showed it to be a huge, distended bladder that contained over 2 liters of urine. Both kidneys were blocked as well and video-urodynamic study confirmed bladder neck obstruction, an exceedingly rare condition. Suzanne was started on intermittent self-catheterization and doxazocin. After three months her kidneys returned to normal. However, she was unable to urinate at all and repeat video-urodynamic study again showed a bladder neck obstruction. I performed a transurethral resection of the bladder neck over five years ago and ever since she's voided to completion, never has day or night incontinence, and her kidneys have continued to be normal.

For men and women with enuresis due to involuntary bladder contractions from neurologic conditions (detrusor hyperreflexia), treatment is much more difficult. For most of the neurologic conditions, there is currently no cure, so the enuresis needs to be treated symptomatically. For some patients, behavior modification is very effective; for others anticholinergic medications (which stop the bladder from contracting involuntarily) may be effective. These topics are discussed in much more detail in Chapters 5 and 17).

Occasionally, people with sphincter abnormalities have enuresis, but this condition is, for practical purposes, always associated with severe daytime incontinence. Treatment of the daytime incontinence cures the enuresis as well.

CONCLUSION

In children, enuresis or bedwetting is very common and usually caused by delayed maturation of the nervous system. With or without treatment, it usually spontaneously gets better. Often, it is the result of a urinary tract infection. Sometimes, though, it can be the sign of a more serious condition such as vesicoureteral reflux, posterior urethral valves, spina bifida, and even spinal cord tumors. For all these reasons, it is important for any child with persistent enuresis to undergo medical evaluation. Urinalysis and culture will determine whether or not there is urinary tract infection and neurologic examination should disclose most neurologic abnormalities. Postvoid residual urine should be measured by ultrasound, and if all else is negative, a voiding diary is most useful in determining the next step in diagnosis and treatment.

On the basis of this evaluation (assuming that urine infection and hematuria have been excluded) it is possible to determine the exact cause of the problem, and in the great majority of people, effective therapy can be instituted. One more thing, though. Many of the conditions that cause adult-onset enuresis also cause silent kidney damage due to high pressures in the bladder. For this reason, it is important to obtain blood tests for kidney function (BUN and creatinine) and a renal ultrasound to be sure that there is not a blockage to the kidney.

8

Stress Incontinence in Women

Margaret is a 47-year-old married homemaker who has a problem with loss of urinary control. That means she is incontinent. At first she merely noticed that her underwear was sometimes damp. That was OK. She could live with that. Then one day, while playing tennis, she lost control. Urine actually dripped down her leg. She was mortified. Her friends must have seen what happened. Well, maybe not. White clothes don't show so much. Maybe that's why people wear white for tennis.

She didn't know what to do or what to say. "Oh my God," she thought. "I can smell the urine myself. I smell. If I smell it, they must be able to smell it." She panicked. She told her friends that she suddenly felt sick and she ran home.

Her clothes were soaked. She called her doctor, but he couldn't come to the telephone. She spoke with the nurse, who cheerfully told her that this is very common. No need to worry. It happens to lots of women and many women just wear pads and it's no big problem at all, but if it really got bad she could have an operation and the doctor would see her right away in three weeks. Three weeks! How could she wait three weeks. What if it happens again. What if someone knows. How could she wear smelly, urine-soaked pads. The nurse said it happens to lots of women. "Who cares; it's happening to me. I don't want to wear pads."

So Margaret suffered in silence for three weeks. In the interim, she began to notice that she sometimes wet herself when she coughed or sneezed. Once in a while she had to change her underwear. It was getting worse! The three weeks were going by awfully slowly. . . .

WHAT'S WRONG WITH MARGARET?

Margaret has a condition called stress urinary incontinence, a condition in which there is involuntary leakage of urine associated with physical activity such as coughing, sneezing, laughing, exercising, and changing positions. In some instances, the condition is so severe that even standing or walking may precipitate the urinary loss. Stress incontinence is due to a weakness of the urinary sphincter. Make a fist with your left hand and stick out your left thumb. Your fist is like the bladder and your thumb is like the urethra. Now put your right hand around your left thumb and squeeze it. Your right hand is like the sphincter. In stress incontinence, the sphincter is weak. It cannot squeeze hard enough to keep urine from leaking out when the pressure inside the bladder gets too high. Stress incontinence is to be distinguished from incontinence due to an overactive bladder. Most people with an overactive bladder have urge incontinence. In people with urge incontinence, the sphincter is usually normal; in fact, it might even be stronger than normal. The problem is that when the bladder contracts involuntarily, you start to urinate involuntarily. Stress incontinence is like a leaky valve; urge incontinence is like an open faucet.

Many people believe that stress incontinence is a consequence of childbirth. Although childbirth is surely an aggravating factor, stress incontinence is due to multiple factors, not just childbirth. The basic abnormality, without which stress incontinence does not occur, is a weakness of the sphincter itself (see Chapter 2 for a more detailed explanation of what the sphincter is and how it works). Normally, no matter how hard you cough or strain or push or exercise, the sphincter stays closed and no urine leaks out. If during such exercise, urine leaks past the sphincter, the sphincter is weakened. This is the basic cause of sphincteric incontinence. However, there is another major aggravating factor, a weakness in the muscular tissues that normally support the bladder and urethra. When these muscles become weakened, the bladder and urethra sag down into the vagina. Figures 1 and 2 show what happens in stress incontinence.

The sagging of the bladder and urethra is called prolapse. When the bladder sags, it is commonly called a "dropped bladder." The medical term for prolapse is *cystocele* (sist-oh-seal). If the urethra drops, it is called a *urethrocele* (you-reeth-ro-seal). When the vaginal muscles are weak, other organs can prolapse as well. Rectal prolapse is called *rectocele* (reck-toh-seal), intestinal prolapse is called *enterocele* (ehn-ter-oh-seal). The uterus and cervix also commonly prolapse, but there is no special name for that; it's just called uterine prolapse.

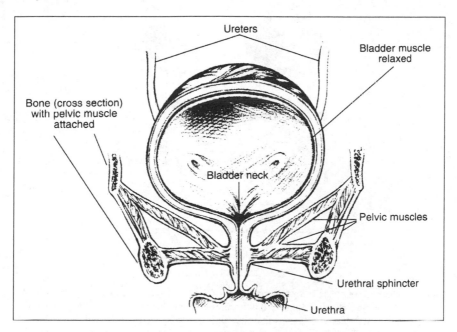

Ureters

Bladder muscle
relaxed

Bone (cross section)
with pelvic muscle
attached

Bladder neck

Pelvic muscles

Urethral sphincter

Urethra

Figure 1. The bladder, urethra, and supporting pelvic muscles. The bladder muscle is normally relaxed and the sphincter muscle is closed except during urination. The bladder and urethra are held in place by the pelvic muscles, which are attached to the bones of the pelvis. No matter how hard you cough or strain or push, the pelvic muscles normally hold things in place and the sphincter stays closed to prevent urine loss. Courtesy of the American Urological Association, Inc., Female Stress Urinary Incontinence Guidelines Panel.

It is commonly thought that prolapse occurs when the vaginal muscles become stretched and weakened during childbirth, but obesity and just the upright position also can result in prolapse. Operations on the vagina, bladder, or urethra can also weaken these supports and cause prolapse and stress incontinence. Creatures that walk on all fours do not develop prolapse and they don't develop stress incontinence. Take a good look at animals that walk on all fours—lions, tigers, elephants, cats, and dogs. No matter how strong or agile they are, they all have potbellies. Well, maybe not potbellies, but their bellies hang down. When a woman walks upright, the equivalent of the belly hanging down is vaginal prolapse, a "hanging down" of the pelvic organs. It occurs because of the way the vagina is shaped. Prolapse doesn't occur in every woman, and maybe exercises to strengthen the pelvic floor muscles help to prevent it, but it does happen to a lot of women and the older you get the more likely it is to happen. But don't worry, there's lots that can be done to prevent it or fix it once it happens.

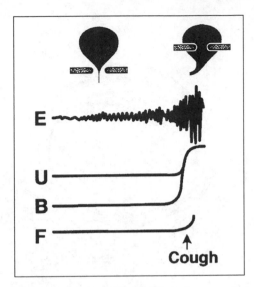

Figure 2. Diagram of stress incontinence. The bladder is shown at the top of the picture. At the left of the tracing, the bladder is full, in normal position, held in place by the pelvic muscles. The horizontal lines on either side of the bladder neck represent the pelvic bones. The pressure in the urethra (U) is greater than the pressure in the bladder (B). The muscular activity of the sphincter (E) is increasing to keep the sphincter closed. There is no leakage of urine. At the right of the tracing, the patient coughed. The urethra (U) opened because the sphincter was weak and the bladder and urethra fell down below the pelvic bones because the pelvic muscles were also weak. The pressure in the bladder (B) increased to the level of the pressure in the urethra (U) and urinary leakage occurred and was measured as uroflow (F).

WHAT CAN BE DONE?

Treatment of incontinence and prolapse is entirely elective. In other words, no treatment is necessary at all unless you find the symptoms bothersome enough. Treatment should be individualized based on your symptoms, goals, and overall medical condition. Some patients with very severe incontinence are quite satisfied if treatment reduces the amount of incontinence to the point where they can manage with absorbent pads. Others are very distressed at the loss of even a few drops of urine and want to be perfectly dry at all times.

Treatment options are varied and run the gamut from absorbent pads, medications, exercises, and electrical stimulation to surgery. Some therapies are of proven efficacy; others are entirely experimental. Surgical treatment, which is widely available, is the most effective, and there have been many scientific studies that evaluate the results of surgery. For this reason, surgical treatment will be discussed first to provide a baseline for comparison with the other forms of therapy.

SURGICAL TREATMENT OF STRESS INCONTINENCE

Although over 125 operations have been designed to treat stress incontinence, they fall into six general categories. All of the operations are based on the same common principles: (1) to restore the support of the bladder and urethra so that they don't fall down again and (2) to provide a kind of backboard against which the urethra is compressed during stress (Figure 3). Take your left hand again and make a bladder. Stick out your left thumb and make a urethra. Now make a V with your right index finger and thumb. I said your right index finger and thumb, not your left! Keep your right hand perfectly still and put your left thumb, parallel to the ground, above the V. Now bang your left thumb (the urethra) against

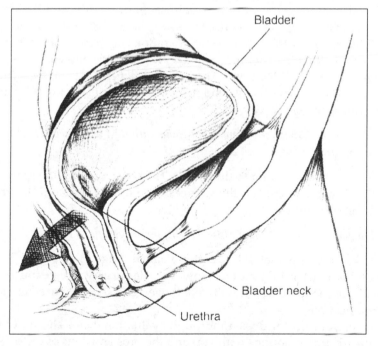

Figure 3. The goal of surgery for stress incontinence is to create a backboard against which the urethra is compressed during stress. The arrow shows the direction that the urethra moves during stress. This is where the backboard should be positioned. Courtesy of the American Urological Association, Inc., Female Stress Urinary Incontinence Guidelines Panel.

the notch of the V (your right thumb and index finger). The V is like a backboard. If your thumb was a soft hollow tube, like the urethra, when it hit the V the urethra (your thumb) would be compressed and no fluid would be able to flow through it.

The six categories of operations for stress incontinence include (1) vaginal suspensions, (2) "needle" suspensions, (3) retropubic suspensions, (4) pubovaginal sling operations, (5) prosthetic sphincters, and (6) peri-urethral injections (I'll explain what these words mean a little later). As you might have guessed, the proponents of each kind of operation think that the operation they do is the best. So, there are actually six best kinds of operations if you believe everything you read. I don't believe everything I read, so first I'll tell you what I think is best.

I think the pubovaginal sling is the best operation because it lasts the longest and has the overall highest cure rate. However, if your doctor isn't experienced in doing this operation, complications can ensue. The retropubic operations are next best because they also last a long time, but they don't work in everyone. The needle suspensions are OK, but they don't seem to last as long, they don't work in as many people, and if your doctor isn't very experienced, there can be very serious complications.

Even though I think that some operations are better than others, the decision about which operation to have (if you've decided to have an operation) is a very difficult one. The decision depends on many factors. It depends on you—your wants and needs, your overall health, the cause of the incontinence, your weight . . .

My weight. What's my weight got to do with it? I don't want to talk about my weight, thank you.

Your weight has a lot to do with it. The fatter you are, the more difficult the surgery, the greater the chances of complications, and the greater the chance of failure.

Do you mean that if I don't lose weight, the surgery won't work?

No. I didn't say that. If I do a pubovaginal sling, it will probably work well and last just as long a time. However, the surgery will be much more difficult for me to do and it will take longer, and there's a greater chance of complications.

After your doctor does a thorough evaluation, he or she should discuss the treatment options with you and the pros and cons of the different surgeries. Your doctor may be very experienced with a lot of operations, but it's not very likely that he or she is experienced with all of them. Most people do some things better than others. In football, some players are

present a clear picture of what life had become like for her. She, like most other IC patients, felt that no one really listened to her, and that the doctors thought it was all in her head.

In this first session the multifaceted behavior modification program was thoroughly explained. She was told that the goals of therapy were (1) to put her back in charge of her bladder, (2) to increase the time between urinations until she was voiding once every four hours or so, and (3) to introduce pain control methods to help rid her of her discomfort. The physiology of pain was reviewed and bladder physiology explained. This is a cognitive therapy in which the patient is an active participant.

Margaret was instructed to keep a voiding diary for 24 hours and to describe her behavior and environment during the next week. Despite living with this problem for so many years, Margaret, like so many other patients, was unaware of just how much fluid she was drinking in a day and did not understand just how many of her behaviors simply reinforced her problem. Seeing things in black and white showed her how "out of control" her life had become and how much room for change there was.

By keeping these records she became an immediate and active participant in investigating her behavior. Let us look at her chart (Figure 1) to better understand how this treatment works. Before each urination she asked herself what degree of discomfort she experienced, on a scale of 0–10, to make her want to urinate. Zero is no discomfort at all; 10 is extreme pain or "bursting," as so many patients seem to say. She put that number in the first column. Although some patients report being at a 9 all of the time, most seem to be around a 5 or 6. They explain to me that they are frightened of letting their discomfort exacerbate to a higher level and remember feeling such intense pain that they usually void more frequently to avoid this discomfort. Other patients void at a 5 or 6 because they are afraid the intensity of discomfort will lead to incontinence. Some have actually wet themselves in a panic, or to relieve pain.

In the next column, Margaret recorded the actual time that she urinated. Before she voided, she asked herself whether she was voiding because she had to (H) or for convenience (C). Convenience means "I don't really have to void now, but I'd better in order to prevent a problem later on or to avoid having to leave an activity." People who do not have a problem with frequency and urgency usually do not have convenience voids. They void when they feel full, and if they can't get to a bathroom right away, they can usually delay for an hour or more. People with a problem have many C voids in a day, and usually know just why this column is included in our chart. Becoming aware of your behaviors will allow you the possibility of changing them. Each convenience void decreases the volume

NAME: Margaret
DATE:

Intensity of pain or urge to void	Time of urination	"C" or "H"	Estimated volume	Actual volume	Events	Oral intake
5	6:00AM	H	300 ml	180 ml	Got up	
5	7:15	H	100 ml	30 ml	Shower	
6	7:45	C	50 ml	30 ml	Breakfast	Coffee
5	8:30	C	50 ml	30 ml		Milk
5	9:20	C	90 ml	30 ml		
6	10:00	H	60 ml	45 ml		
7	10:35	C	50 ml	30 ml		
6	11:15	H	20 ml	30 ml		Soda
7	12:00 PM	H	60 ml	45 ml		
5	1:10	C	60 ml	30 ml	Lunch	Soda
7	1:30	C	150 ml	90 ml		
6	1:40	C	10 ml	90 ml		
6	2:55	H	120 ml	60 ml		
4	3:30	C	90 ml	120 ml		
6	4:30	H	60 ml	30 ml		
5	5:45	H	50 ml	30 ml		
4	7:00	C	100 ml	60 ml	Dinner	Water
4	9:00	C	150 ml	90 ml		Wine
5	11:00	C	120 ml	60 ml		
5	2:00AM	H	120 ml	120 ml		

Figure 1. Margaret's voiding diary. Intensity is recorded on a scale of 0–10; 0 indicates no pain or urge, 10 indicates extreme pain or urge. "C" = voiding out of convenience; "H" = voiding because of urge.

your bladder could be holding. It reinforces the behavior we would like to eliminate and forever keeps the problem on your mind.

In the next column Margaret wrote down the amount of urine that she thought she would void. At first, her guesses were very inaccurate, but in time she was able to estimate with a high degree of accuracy. There is a very important reason for this column. At the beginning of treatment most patients void very frequently and for different reasons—but usually not in response to a full bladder. They void preventively, in response to burning, pressure, pelvic discomfort, for convenience, etc. If you predict and then measure over an 8- to 12-week period, one goal is that your predictions will eventually be in line with what you measure and that you will learn the difference in sensation between 30 ml (1 oz.) and 250 ml (nearly 8 oz.). This is an essential part of the behavioral program that helps you eventually to void only when the bladder is full, overriding other sensations that might make you want to urinate.

Next, Margaret recorded the amount of urine that she actually voided. Most people use a measuring cup from the kitchen, but you can use any container that is convenient. While at work, if you prefer not to carry a measuring cup, use disposable Styrofoam or paper cups and throw them away.

In the next column Margaret made observations about her voiding, including any circumstances that she thought may have brought about the pattern of voiding or the actual discomfort. People can become excellent observers of what circumstances make a situation worse or better. You might notice that you have a very slow stream and urinate in a stop–start fashion at first (because you try to void with such a small amount in your bladder). As you improve and are able to hold larger and larger amounts in your bladder (and urinate larger volumes at one time) you'll notice that the stream is stronger and more continuous.

Besides having a slow stream, Margaret observed that she would stop the stream in anticipation of the burning that she always felt as soon as she'd start to urinate. She also noted that when she was anxious her symptoms worsened. In the last column she recorded the time and amount of her oral intake of food and liquid.

On the basis of her charts, the therapist tailored a treatment program for Margaret. From column 2, you can see that she voided an average of once every hour, with a volume of 90 ml (3 oz.). The largest volume she voided was only 180 ml (6 oz.) and she sometimes voided only an ounce (30 ml). She voided four to five times a night, which was not surprising since she voided so frequently in small volumes during the day. Some people, however, void frequently during the day and for some reason are able to sleep through the night holding a larger quantity of urine.

Margaret usually rated the intensity of her urge to urinate at 6–8, but with this urge, her voided volumes ranged from 30 ml (1 oz.) to 180 ml (6 oz.). All those volumes felt the same to her. She drank an average of 35 ounces of fluid a day, although reported that when traveling she drank as little as possible.

My goal for Margaret was that by gradually increasing the time between urinations and keeping her drinking consistent each day, she would gradually be able to hold more and more urine until she was voiding only once every three to four hours with volumes of 150 ml (5 oz.) or more.

Some patients report an ease and diminution in the burning symptom as their volumes increase, and the urine is more dilute. Confidence in being able to delay micturition and eliminate convenience voids comes only very gradually over time. This is why the time intervals between urinations are increased only very gradually. Sometimes I advise people to delay urination for only 5 minutes, sometimes as much as 30 minutes, depending on the individual. Most people can delay micturition by 15 minutes without panicking or becoming anxious. When you have experienced high levels of discomfort (from burning, pain, etc.) you are often afraid to wait to void. Yet, if you remember back before your symptoms developed, you would often feel an urge to urinate, not be able to get to a bathroom, and have to delay often by as much as 15 minutes to an hour. Usually the urge increases, then seems to diminish, either because you forget about it or the bladder quiets down at that volume, and then you void when it is convenient.

As you see behaviors changing, feel more in control and more confident, you become less anxious and less focused on the symptoms in delaying micturition. The goal of this program is to have you lead as normal a life as possible without this symptom interfering with your day-to-day life. There are no general rules about what to eat or what to drink. You do not have to avoid different foods or drinks; you do not have to be on a special diet. However, if, because of your record keeping, you have found that something bothers your bladder, then avoid it. For many people, certain food or drink, such as caffeine, alcohol, chocolate, salt, or spicy foods, seems to bring on symptoms. If this is the case with you, they should be eliminated from your diet. Once your bladder symptoms have improved and you have reached your goal, these foods can be reintroduced, one at a time, to test the effect on your symptoms. Then you can decide if you want to continue eating or drinking these things.

Some people drink large quantities of fluid "to cleanse the bladder" because they think it is healthy to do so. Health books tell you to drink as much as eight 10-ounce glasses per day; doctors tell you it's good to drink a lot. Many diets stress a high fluid intake. Jane, a 28-year-old secretary, was on a high-fluid diet. By constantly filling up on fluids, she felt less hungry, and, indeed, she lost a lot of weight. But she also voided every 30 minutes during the day and was up every hour at night to urinate. She had always suffered from urinary frequency, but when she went on a weight reduction diet, she increased her fluid intake to more than 2 quarts per day (2 liters) and her frequency and discomfort began to interfere with her daily life. She began behavior modification and did a voiding diary and found that she was uncomfortable at bladder volumes of about 120 ml (4 oz.). After a simple behavioral program lasting four weeks, she decreased her daily fluid intake to an average of 1500 ml (1½ qt.) and increased her bladder capacity to an average void of 240 ml (8 oz.) and was voiding every four hours. Jane was a perfect candidate for behavior modification and soon learned that by trying to control one problem (her weight) she had brought on another (frequency of urination).

Almost all people with IC have nocturia (urination that takes place during the sleeping hours). Most of the time this occurs because the bladder simply can't hold enough urine to permit a full night's sleep—bladder filling hurts too much and wakes them up to urinate. Some people, though, unconsciously make the situation worse. They drink normally during the day, but in the evening, when eating and relaxing, they drink more, and that compounds the underlying problem of painful bladder filling. It is only by diary keeping and looking at the results that you get a clear picture of what needs to be changed.

The behaviors that cause symptoms are observable and measurable. Both you and your therapist can assess the problem and see the improvements and the effectiveness of treatment. Your own involvement and participation is an essential part of behavior modification. All of the strategies utilized in this program are individualized to your particular needs, based on observations made in diary keeping. Techniques that are helpful in one patient may actually be harmful for another.

The most basic tool of behavior modification is called the bladder drill, which is simply a gradual and purposeful increase in the time interval between urinations. Over the weeks of therapy, bladder drill will be used to control frequency of urination and the bladder will get used to holding increased volumes of urine. During this time, in addition to the weekly voiding diary, the patient is asked to keep a daily notebook, keeping track not only of his or her voiding intervals but also activities, circumstances, and any feelings that might be relevant to voiding intervals. Most patients complain of pelvic pressure, discomfort, pain, and burning; a simple bladder drill is often not the solution to these pain syndromes. Strategies for controlling pain must be taught and incorporated into the program. Further, alleviating the depression associated with these refractory bladder symptoms is an essential part of the program. Another integral part of the program is to increase your physical activity. Exercise stimulates endorphin production, which can give an enhanced sense of well-being, and help fight pain, each of which will lead to greater control over your body. Additionally, deep-breathing exercises, transcendental meditation, total body relaxation, and guided imagery are all techniques that can be incorporated into your program. Stress can exacerbate discomfort. Although you certainly cannot eliminate all stress from your life, you can learn to recognize your own unique stress response, become more sensitive and aware of the situations that may trigger it, and learn to control it and react to it in a positive way. The therapist can help you develop strategies that work for you, and take into consideration the physiological, social, and psychological components that can be altered by the behavioral process.

Behavior modification is effective in the majority of my patients, but not everyone derives benefit and not everyone agrees to even undergo that form of treatment. Other treatments include oral and intravesical medications and hydrodistension. These are all discussed in the next few sections.

Oral Medications

A great number of oral medications have been used to treat interstitial cystitis. These include antibiotics, antihistamines, anticholinergics, calcium channel blockers, muscle relaxants, steroids, tranquilizers and antidepressants, pain medications, and even narcotics. Most of these medications have proved ineffective. In my judgment, antibiotics should only be used when there is an infection and despite the frustrating chronicity and pain of IC, narcotic pain medications should not be used except for particularly severe, acute flare-ups. Amitriptyline (Elavil) is a tricyclic antidepressant that has been found to be effective in many patients and for many patients has become a mainstay of treatment. Pentosan polysulfate sodium (Elmiron), an analgesic, has recently been approved by the FDA and is said to work in about one-third of patients.

Intravesical Instillations

Intravesical instillation of medications to treat interstitial cystitis has been performed for at least three decades. The technique is quite simple. A small catheter is passed through the urethra into the bladder and the medication, in the form of a liquid, is injected through the catheter into the bladder. The catheter is removed and the medication remains in the bladder until you urinate approximately 20 minutes later. It is thought that contact of the medication directly with the bladder wall is responsible for the treatment effect. There are a number of formulations used for intravesical instillations. The most common medication used is DMSO (dimethyl sulfoxide). This is often mixed with other medications including steroids, heparin (a blood thinner), lidocaine (an anesthetic) and sodium bicarbonate (to reduce acidity). Intravesical instillations are usually required at weekly or monthly intervals and usually require 6 to 12 treatments. In my judgment, this treatment is effective in less than half of patients. Treatment is time consuming and in some patients, passage of the catheter and instillation of the medication is uncomfortable. Some patients are also unable to hold the urine for the required 20 minutes or so because of bladder pain. Finally, there is a small chance of bladder infection after each catheterization.

Hydrodistension of the Bladder

If medications and behavior modification fail, hydrodistension of the bladder can be considered. It is said to be effective in as many as 50% of people with IC. It is performed by simply filling the bladder under pressure and leaving it distended for a period of time. It can be done under general anesthesia for 5 or 10 minutes and that is probably a reasonable thing to do. However, a more effective procedure is to distend the bladder under spinal or epidural anesthesia using a specially designed balloon catheter that is inserted into the bladder and inflated with X-ray contrast material while the pressure in the bladder is being monitored. Fluid is added to or removed from the balloon, keeping the pressure just below the blood pressure. In this fashion, the bladder is gradually stretched for approximately four hours. At the end of the procedure, the catheter is removed and another catheter is placed overnight. The catheter is removed in the morning. The urine is often bloody for a day or so but you are generally able to leave the hospital the morning after the hydrodistension.

Complications are very unlikely. Occasionally a bladder infection is encountered and rarely the bladder can be ruptured during the procedure. As awful as this sounds, bladder rupture is generally a mild problem that is treated only with a Foley catheter and antibiotics for about a week.

WHAT IS THE CAUSE OF INTERSTITIAL CYSTITIS?

Despite an enormous amount of research into the cause of IC, no one knows for sure. There are a number of very logical explanations, but none has been supported by consistent research findings. Dr. Lowell Parsons, a urologist in San Diego, California, and one of the pioneering researchers in this area, believes that there is an increased permeability of the bladder wall to certain substances that cause the disease. Normally, there is a layer of proteins called *glycosaminoglycans* that bind with water and form a protective coating to the bladder wall that prevents bacteria from sticking to it and prevents chemicals from getting into it. Dr. Parsons believes that this layer is reduced in patients with IC, sensitizing the bladder to substances (like bacteria or chemicals) in the urine that cause the symptoms.

Another popular theory is that there is an abnormality of one of the cells in the bladder wall called the mast cell. In 20–65% of patients with IC there is *mastocytosis*—an increased number of mast cells in the wall of the bladder. The mast cells contain little packets called granules that secrete different chemicals. Some of these chemicals, particularly one called histamine, are nocioceptive, which means that they cause pain. However, mastocytosis commonly occurs from inflammation of any cause and could very well be the result, rather than the cause, of IC.

Many other theories have been proposed by researchers, but none have enough supporting evidence to make them convincing to the scientific community. Some believe that IC is an autoimmune disease like systemic lupus. Others believe that there is a mysterious toxic substance in the urine that causes the symptoms. Still others believe that it is a manifestation of an overactivity of the sympathetic nervous system known as reflex sympathetic dystrophy. As you probably realize by now, though, at the present time, the cause is pretty much unknown.

CONCLUSION

Interstitial cystitis is an uncommon condition that afflicts about 250,000–500,000 Americans, over 90% of whom are women. The cause is unknown. The most important aspect of the evaluation for this condition is to have a proper checkup to be sure that the symptoms are not caused by a simple problem like a urinary tract infection and to exclude more serious conditions such as bladder cancer. Treatment is empirical, and there are many different therapeutic regimens, but in expert hands, treatment is successful in the majority of patients.

12

Difficulty Urinating and Urinary Retention

John is a 49-year-old computer programmer. He was at the stadium watching a baseball game with his family when he experienced a normal urge to urinate. He waited for about a half hour, then went to the bathroom. There was a line at the men's room, so he waited and the urge got much stronger. When he finally got to the stall, he couldn't urinate. The discomfort became worse and worse and he became self-conscious about holding up the line. He panicked and began to perspire. He began to push and strain and finally a few drops came out, then some more urine came out, then he voided with a very thin stream. Later that night at home, he voided normally again. Or so he thought.

He saw his family doctor and everything checked out fine, but he sought the advice of a urologist. A flow test showed that his "normal" urination was, in fact, very weak, and that he retained a lot of urine in his bladder after urinating. This caused a backup of urine that had resulted in kidney damage. He was found to have bladder neck obstruction, a form of blockage in the urethra, and he underwent a small operation (bladder neck incision). Afterward, the kidneys came back to normal and he urinated normally, with no residual urine.

Diana is a 34-year-old married lawyer. She's had an increasing problem with frequency and urgency of urination, having to rush to the bathroom to urinate, sometimes even in the middle of court. Recently, though, when she has gotten to the bathroom, only a few drops come out and sometimes she is unable to urinate at all. She was checked by her doctor, and it turned out that she had a bladder infection and was urinating so frequently that there was never very much in her bladder. She was treated with antibiotics and the symptoms resolved.

Pat, a 53-year-old married housewife, had become aware that her urinary stream was always weak and intermittent. It had been that way for at least 20 years, but she never paid any attention to it. Whenever she urinated, she had to sit and wait. A few drops would come out, then a weak stream, then a few more drops. She would get up, leave the bathroom, get another urge and return, and the same thing would happen. On routine gynecological examination, her doctor felt a mass in her abdomen. An ultrasound was done and she was found to have an enormous bladder. She was catheterized for over 2 liters, that's over 70 ounces! After the catheter was removed, she was not able to urinate at all. She underwent an extensive evaluation and was found to have a rare blockage of the urethra. She underwent corrective surgery and she is now completely normal.

Danny is a 35-year-old salesman. He was never, under any circumstances, able to urinate anyplace else but in his own home, in his own bathroom. It had been like that for as long as he could remember. He planned his life around the proximity of his own bathroom. He worked near home and when he had to urinate, he went home. If he tried to urinate in any other bathroom, he simply could not do so. He'd push and strain; he'd try to relax, but nothing would ever come out.

After an extensive evaluation, he was found to have a learned voiding dysfunction, which is like a bad habit. Danny had subconscious fears about urinating and every time he would try to void outside of his own bathroom, he would unconsciously contract his sphincter and hold the urine back. After a two-month course of behavior modification he was voiding in public bathrooms without difficulty and had taken a new job that required extensive travel.

Eric, a 72-year-old retired waiter, always had to push and strain to start urination and there was a long delay before he could start. When he finally voided, the stream was very thin and weak. He saw a urologist who told him that he had a prostate blockage. He was treated with medication and now he is fine.

As you can see, all of these people had similar symptoms, but in each case, the cause and the treatment were very different. The symptoms of difficulty urinating are hesitancy and weak stream. Hesitancy means a delay in starting micturition. You get an urge to go to the bathroom and stand or sit there and nothing comes out. Some people push with their abdominal muscles and strain to try to force the urine out; others close their eyes, try to relax, and let the urine come out by itself. Still others have found that if they lean forward or sit backward or stand or sit, it's easier to void. Some people tap or push on their lower abdomen; some listen to the sound of running water.

A weak stream may be a very thin stream or it may be a dribbling or interrupted stream that stops and starts many times before you're finished. If you are like John, you might have been born with a weak stream and not even know that you have one.

WHAT CAUSES DIFFICULT URINATION?

There are only two basic causes of difficulty urinating—either a blockage to the flow of urine through the urethra (like John, Pat, and Eric) or a weakened bladder. The bladder muscle may become so weakened that it cannot contract strongly enough or long enough to empty itself or there may be damage to the nervous system making it impossible for the bladder to contract at all or for you to give it the signal to contract. Another cause of difficulty urinating, which is not really a pathological condition, is insufficient urine in the bladder for you to urinate. This is the problem Diana had, but in her case it was due to infection. If the bladder has only a small amount of urine, voiding is very difficult even for normal people. Finally, there may be a learned voiding dysfunction—a bad habit, like Danny had.

A complete list of the most common causes of difficulty urinating is found in Table 1. The causes in men and women, however, are very different. In men, the most common cause, by far, is a blockage due to the prostate. In most men with prostatic blockage, the bladder works normally; in fact, it often becomes stronger than normal because of the blockage. The reason that these men have difficulty urinating is because it takes a much higher pressure to force the urine out of a urethra that is partially blocked by the prostate. This subject is discussed in great detail in the next chapter.

In women, it is not so obvious what the common causes are. In my experience the most common cause is trying to urinate when there is an insufficient amount of urine in the bladder.

What difference does it make how much urine there is in the bladder?

Remember, the bladder is a muscular sac that holds urine. In order to urinate, the bladder muscle must contract, squeezing out the urine through the urethra. Every muscle contracts best at a certain degree of

Table 1. Causes of Difficulty Urinating

A. Bladder causes:
1. Damage to the bladder nerves (neurogenic bladder)
   a. Spinal cord injury
   b. Multiple sclerosis
   c. Diabetes mellitus
   d. Herniated (ruptured) disc
2. Weak bladder
   a. Due to urethral obstruction (blockage)
   b. Idiopathic (no known cause)
3. Inability to voluntarily make the bladder contract to start urination (initiate the micturition reflex)
   a. Damage to the bladder nerves (neurologic)—stroke, spinal cord injury, multiple sclerosis
   b. Psychological (psychogenic)
4. Too little urine in the bladder
   a. Hypersensitive bladder—urinary tract infection, interstitial cystitis, prostatic obstruction, bladder and prostate cancer
   b. Detrusor overactivity—idiopathic detrusor instability, stroke, spinal cord injury, prostatic obstruction, multiple sclerosis
B. Blockage in the urethra
1. Vesical neck obstruction
2. Prostatic obstruction
3. Urethral stricture
4. Learned voiding dysfunction

stretch. Imagine throwing a baseball. You stretch your arm backwards, way past your ear and then, when it is as far back as possible, the muscles of your arm contract forcibly propelling your arm (and the ball) forward. Now imagine that you were told to throw the baseball as far as you could, but you were not allowed to move your hand past your nose. You wouldn't be able to throw it very far because the muscles in your arm never stretched to their optimal length for throwing. In order for the bladder to contract well, it, too, has to be stretched to near capacity. If you try to urinate before then, it will be much more difficult and you may not be able to urinate at all until it fills (stretches) more.

What would cause a woman to try to urinate when there isn't very much in her bladder?

The causes are listed in the table, but I can explain a little better here. The two most common causes of this are a hypersensitive bladder and an overactive bladder. A hypersensitive bladder is one in which the bladder becomes more and more uncomfortable as the bladder fills with urine. The discomfort may be due to obvious causes such as urinary tract infection (like Diana had) or a bladder stone or bladder cancer, all of which cause inflammation of the bladder wall. Or there may be an abnormality of the bladder wall itself so that bladder filling is painful. There may be a toxic or noxious substance in the urine itself that causes pain. (These topics are discussed in detail in Chapter 11.)

An overactive bladder is one that contracts involuntarily. When the bladder contracts involuntarily one of two things happens; you either get a sudden urge to urinate and then contract your sphincter to prevent incontinence or, if you are unable to do that, you lose control of your urine and wet yourself. People with involuntary bladder contractions may experience these urges to urinate for no obvious or conscious reason at all (but in fact they are due to involuntary bladder contractions). Involuntary contractions may occur anytime, with any amount of urine in the bladder. So you might be sitting down, comfortably reading, and you'll get a sudden urge to urinate (due to an involuntary bladder contraction). There isn't very much urine in your bladder, but it feels like there is because of the bladder contraction. You get up and go to the bathroom, but by the time you get there, the involuntary contraction has subsided. You try to urinate, but there isn't much in the bladder and you push and strain and only a few drops come out.

There are many causes of these involuntary contractions. They are subdivided into neurologic and nonneurologic causes. The nonneurologic causes are much more common, but once again, the causes are different in men and women. In women, most are idiopathic (of unknown origin) but they are also commonly associated with stress incontinence (see Chapter 8) and also with advancing age and estrogen deficiency. In men they are most often associated with prostatic obstruction (Chapter 13). The neurologic causes affect both sexes and include stroke, Parkinson's disease, multiple sclerosis, diabetes mellitus, and spinal cord injury (see Chapter 17).

I have these symptoms, but they really don't bother me very much. Do I need to see a doctor anyway?

It's very important to have the symptoms checked out to be sure that there is not a serious underlying condition causing them—bladder or prostate cancer, for example. Fortunately, such serious life-threatening conditions are not common. Once you've been evaluated, treatment is entirely elective unless the underlying condition is one that poses a threat to your health.

COLLEGE OF THE SEQUOIAS
LIBRARY

DIAGNOSTIC EVALUATION

The purpose of the diagnostic evaluation is to determine the cause of your symptoms and to determine the need for treatment. As always, the evaluation begins with a history and physical examination. A urine sample should be obtained to check for infection and blood in the urine. If infection is found, you will be treated with antibiotics. If there is blood in the urine you should have a complete evaluation for that, including cystoscopy and X ray of your kidneys. If the urinalysis and culture are negative, you should have a uroflow and measurement of postvoid residual urine. The uroflow measures how forcibly the urine comes out and the postvoid residual urine determines how well you empty your bladder. Both of these tests are usually done during the same visit. Neither is invasive and neither hurts. The uroflow is obtained by having you urinate into a funnel-shaped receptacle at the bottom of which is an electronic device to measure the rate of urine flow. The postvoid residual urine is estimated by placing an ultrasonic probe on your lower abdomen over the bladder. Postvoid residual urine may also be measured by passing a catheter through the urethra into the bladder, but this is an invasive test that could be a little painful and could cause a urinary tract infection. Whenever possible, I think it is better to measure with ultrasound rather than a catheter. Finally, you should keep a voiding diary for at least 24 hours recording the time and amount of each urination.

On the basis of this preliminary evaluation, your doctor should be able to develop a working diagnosis—a listing of the most probable causes of your symptoms as outlined in Table 1. In many cases the diagnosis will be obvious and you may proceed directly with treatment. However, if it is necessary to determine whether the symptoms are caused by a weak bladder or a blockage, further testing will be necessary. You will need to undergo urodynamic testing as discussed in Chapter 4. There are a number of different tests and combinations of tests that go under the generic heading of urodynamics, but in this case it is important that you undergo multichannel urodynamics with (at least) synchronous detrusor pressure/uroflow determination. Optimally, you should undergo video-urodynamics. After urodynamic study, the chances are that your doctor will have a diagnosis and should offer you treatment options based on the cause.

A listing of the possible treatments, based on the cause of difficulty urinating, is listed in Table 2.

When difficulty urinating is caused by damage to the bladder nerves, in most cases there is little that can be done to reverse the condition and most patients who require treatment will be advised to do self intermittent catheterization (discussed below). Occasionally there may be a remediable condition, such as a ruptured disc that remits after treatment. Further,

Table 2. Treatment of Difficulty Urinating

Cause	Treatment
Damage to bladder nerves	Treat underlying neurologic condition
	Intermittent self-catheterization
Weak bladder	Treat coexisting blockage
	Intermittent self-catheterization
Loss of voluntary bladder control	Treat underlying neurologic condition
	Behavior modification
Hypersensitive bladder	Treat underlying condition
	Behavior modification
Overactive bladder	Treat underlying neurologic condition
	Treat coexisting blockage
Blockage in the urethra	Treat blockage

some neurologic conditions such as multiple sclerosis have a tendency to remit and the bladder problem may spontaneously subside.

If intermittent catheterization is not possible it may be necessary to use an indwelling catheter. This is a catheter that is passed through the urethra and stays in the bladder continuously. The other end of the catheter is attached to tubing and then to a plastic drainage bag that stores the urine, which is periodically emptied into a toilet. The catheter itself should be changed about once every two to four weeks.

If the problem is a weakened bladder there are two possibilities. Intermittent catheterization is the mainstay of treatment, but many men will respond favorably to empirical treatment (trial and error) for prostatic obstruction, such as alpha-adrenergic blocking medications, or prostatic surgery. In women, surgery is ill advised unless a definite blockage has been diagnosed, and this is extraordinarily uncommon.

If the bladder does not contract at all (detrusor areflexia) and the cause is a neurologic one, there is little alternative to self intermittent catheterization. However, if the cause is a learned voiding dysfunction, behavior modification may be effective.

In patients with a hypersensitive or overactive bladder, treatment of the underlying cause is almost always effective in relieving the voiding symptoms. The most dramatic response to treatment, though, is seen after prostate surgery in men who suffer from prostatic obstruction (see Chapter 13).

SELF INTERMITTENT CATHETERIZATION

Intermittent catheterization may be used as a temporary means of managing your bladder while you are awaiting other therapies, or it may be used as definitive treatment over a lifetime. Except in the most unusual of circumstances, you should do intermittent catheterization yourself and not rely on a nurse, aide, or family member. If you do the catheterization yourself, it is called self intermittent catheterization (SIC). SIC is generally meant to replace normal urination, but sometimes, particularly if you are unable to urinate after surgery, you should try to urinate first, then catheterize yourself. Most authorities agree that when doing SIC, there is no need for sterile technique; there is no need for gloves; there is no need for antiseptic solutions. All that is necessary is a catheter and some lubrication to allow easy insertion of the catheter into the urethra. The procedure is simple and painless. You go into a bathroom, sit or stand, put a dab of lubricant on the tip of the catheter, and insert the catheter into the penis and through the urethra into the bladder in men (Figure 1) or into the vaginal opening of the urethra in women (Figure 2). Once the catheter is inside the bladder urine will begin to flow out and you should keep the catheter in place until the urine stops flowing. You may assist the urine flow by pushing down on your abdomen; this will cause the urine to come out faster. In general, within the limits of comfort, the larger the size of the catheter the easier it is to insert and the faster the urine comes out. For that reason relatively larger sizes (16–18 french) are more desirable than smaller catheters (8–14 french).

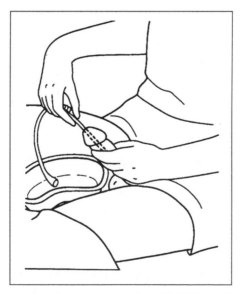

Figure 1. Intermittent catheterization in a man. From M. B. Chancellor & J. G. Blaivas, *Practical Neuro-Urology—Genitourinary Complications in Neurologic Disease,* Butterworth-Heinemann, Boston, 1995, with permission.

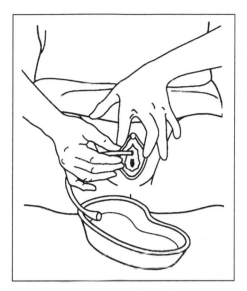

Figure 2. Intermittent catheterization in a woman. From M. B. Chancellor & J. G. Blaivas, *Practical Neuro-Urology—Genitourinary Complications in Neurologic Disease,* Butterworth-Heinemann, Boston, 1995, with permission.

To most people who are unfamiliar with the technique, it seems barbarous and unhygienic, and something that they would never want to do. In fact, it has proven to be one of the most useful treatment modalities to emerge over the last two to three decades. For the overwhelming majority of patients, passage of the catheter is painless and poses little inconvenience. For the patient who is hopelessly incontinent or unable to urinate at all, it is a salvation. Intermittent catheterization may be used as a temporary measure to treat patients recovering from surgery or awaiting surgery, or it may be used as definitive treatment.

There are three basic conditions for which intermittent catheterization is indicated: first, in patients whose bladder simply doesn't contract because of either nerve or muscle damage; second, for patients with severe obstruction; and finally, for patients who have incontinence due to involuntary bladder contractions in whom it is desirable to abolish the contractions with either medicine or surgery and then empty the bladder with the catheter.

CONCLUSION

Difficulty urinating and urinary retention have two general causes—weak or absent bladder contractions and urethral blockage. Less commonly there may be learned voiding dysfunction, which can be likened to a bad habit. Finally, some people try to urinate when the bladder is insufficiently filled either because of a false message or because the bladder contracts involuntarily.

In almost all patients an accurate diagnosis can be obtained by performing a proper evaluation consisting of history and physical examination, urinalysis and urine culture, voiding diary, uroflow and postvoid residual determination, and, finally, urodynamics.

No matter what the cause, there is almost always an acceptable and effective treatment. When there is blockage in men, prostate surgery is nearly always successful, but there are many alternative approaches including medications and minimally invasive surgery. Learned voiding dysfunctions are best treated with behavior modification, and detrusor overactivity is treated by eliminating the cause of the overactive bladder. When all else fails—almost exclusively in people with serious neurologic conditions—intermittent self-catheterization is the treatment of choice and for most is a godsend, enabling them to resume a nearly normal lifestyle.

13

Benign Prostate Problems

There is probably a very good reason why men have prostate glands, but as yet, no one has figured out why. The prostate gland seems to be much more of a benefit to urologists (it accounts for as much as half of their income) than it is to the person in whose body the prostate resides. The prostate is a specialized gland that surrounds the male urethra near the opening to the bladder (Figure 1). It produces secretions that are mixed with sperm during ejaculation.

At birth, the prostate is proportionately very small. It remains small until approximately age 40, at which time there is a gradual increase in its size to perhaps the size of a walnut. This increase in size occurs because the prostate cells actually get larger and more numerous. This condition is called benign prostatic hyperplasia, commonly known as BPH. By age 80, approximately 80% of men have BPH. BPH is often associated with lower urinary tract symptoms, and it can cause bladder and kidney problems, as discussed below, but for most men it is more of a nuisance than a threat to their health. Although many men with BPH develop prostate cancer, BPH does not cause cancer.

The exact cause of BPH is not known, but many other facts about it are known. First, it only occurs when the male hormone, called testosterone, is present in the bloodstream. Testosterone is produced by the testicles. It is actually one of the breakdown products of testosterone, called dihydrotestosterone, or DHT, that is responsible for BPH. If the testicles are removed during childhood, thereby removing the major source of testosterone, BPH does not occur. You might not want to do that to your son, though. For that reason, most men, if they live long enough, do get BPH.

The other major cause of prostatic enlargement is cancer of the prostate. If you're a male, and lucky enough to live to an old age, you'll

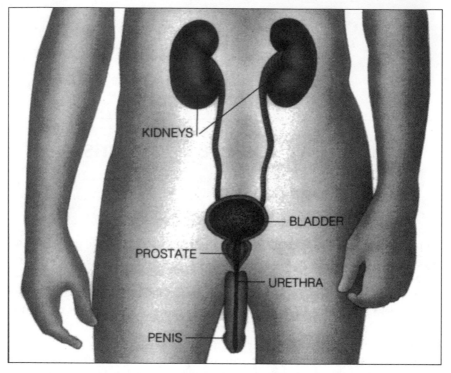

Figure 1. Location of the prostate gland. Courtesy of American Foundation of Urologic Diseases.

probably get that too. By age 80 more than half of men, whether they know it or not, have prostate cancer. Prostate cancer will be discussed in detail in Chapter 14.

LOWER URINARY TRACT SYMPTOMS IN MEN (PROSTATISM)

Accompanying the growth of the prostate (whether it's benign or malignant), many patients develop lower urinary tract symptoms (LUTS) that are commonly known as prostatism. However, the word *prostatism* conveys the message that the symptoms are due to the prostate. Since this is not always the case, we prefer to use the phrase LUTS. LUTS is a group of symptoms that consists of the following:

1. Weak urinary stream.
2. Hesitancy (a delay before urination starts).
3. Intermittency (an interrupted urinary stream).

4. Frequency of urination.
5. Urgency of urination (an uncomfortable, painful feeling in the lower abdomen and at the tip of the penis that makes you rush to the bathroom).
6. Nocturia (being awakened at night because of the need to urinate).
7. Urge incontinence (loss of urinary control because of a strong urge to urinate).
8. Postvoid dribbling (a dribbling loss of urine that occurs immediately after urination).

There are four basic causes of LUTS:

1. An obstruction or blockage to the flow of urine through the urethra.
2. A weakened bladder muscle that cannot contract strongly enough.
3. Detrusor instability (involuntary contractions of the bladder).
4. A hypersensitivity of the bladder that gives you the feeling that you have to urinate even when there is not much urine in the bladder.

A man with LUTS may have one or more of these underlying conditions in any combination. Most importantly, the symptoms of prostatism are not always due to BPH; they may be mimicked by a number of other conditions, including urinary tract infection, cancer of the prostate, cancer of the bladder, neurogenic bladder (an abnormality of the nerve supply to the bladder), infections and inflammations of the prostate, and bladder or kidney stones. The only way to determine what is causing the symptoms is to undergo a proper urologic evaluation as discussed below.

WHEN SHOULD I GO TO THE DOCTOR AND WHAT SHOULD THE DOCTOR DO?

An enlarged prostate is often discovered on a routine annual checkup during rectal examination. In the great majority of men, enlargement of the prostate is due to BPH, but with or without BPH, there is a possibility of prostate cancer. As mentioned, BPH does not cause prostate cancer, but many men with BPH develop prostate cancer. If your internist or general practitioner suspects a prostate abnormality on examination, or if you have LUTS, he should obtain a urinalysis. If there is blood in the urine, if there is a urinary tract infection, or if there is a suspicion of cancer on the examination of the prostate, you should be referred to a urologist. If the urinalysis shows infection, a urine culture should be done and you should be treated with antibiotics.

If there is no blood in the urine and there is no urinary tract infection and there is no suspicion of cancer, your doctor should discuss his findings with you and determine whether any further evaluation or treatment is necessary. This is most appropriately done at a second visit after the results of the urine and blood tests are available. In addition, blood tests (BUN and creatinine) should be done to check how well your kidneys are working because, rarely, prostatic obstruction can lead to kidney damage.

How do you know if you need further evaluation and treatment? You need more tests and treatment if (1) you think that your symptoms are bothersome enough to warrant treatment or (2) your doctor has found an abnormality that requires further evaluation. This brings up an area of controversy. Most doctors think that if a patient does not consider the symptoms bad enough to warrant treatment, the evaluation ends then and there, provided that the examination and lab tests did not disclose something that needs to be treated. Other doctors believe that in certain instances, a renal and bladder ultrasound should be performed, and I agree. The purpose of these tests is to be sure that the way you are urinating has not harmed your bladder or kidneys. The blood tests will determine whether or not the kidneys are working normally, but they cannot tell whether one kidney is abnormal and the other one is taking over its function. In addition, the blood tests can't tell whether or not there is an obstruction or a blockage that has already begun to damage the kidney but not so severely to cause the blood tests to be abnormal. On the other hand, a perfectly normal ultrasound is reassuring and thus both you and your doctor know that it is okay to withhold any further therapy for as long as you are comfortable doing so.

WHEN TO SEE A UROLOGIST

A urologist is both a physician and surgeon who specializes in, among other things, disorders of the lower urinary tract. In men, the lower urinary tract consists of the bladder, prostate, sphincter, and urethra. You should see a urologist if you develop persistent LUTS.

What do you mean by persistent? Is two days persistent?

"Persistent" depends on how abruptly the symptoms begin. If you feel perfectly well one minute and the next, you feel like you have to urinate, but go to the bathroom and nothing comes out, and if that persists for more than five or six hours, you should call or see a doctor. If you've seen a urologist before, you should call him. If you can't see a urologist, you should see either your primary care doctor or go to an emergency room. These symptoms could be the beginning of urinary retention, a urinary tract infection, a kidney stone, or even more serious conditions such as prostate cancer.

If you have a more gradual onset of symptoms—for example, a gradually increasing frequency and urgency of urination or a weakening urinary stream—you may wait weeks or months before seeing a urologist. Of course it's still necessary to see a primary care physician to be sure that there are no signs of infection or blood in the urine. There are a number of warning signs that make consulting with a urologist more urgent. These include (1) severe LUTS that do not respond to treatment by your primary care doctor; (2) a suspicion of prostate cancer, either because of an abnormality on prostate exam or an elevated prostate-specific antigen (PSA) (as shown on your blood tests); (3) elevated postvoid residual urine (incomplete emptying of the bladder after urinating); (4) a very weak urinary stream; (5) blood in the urine (hematuria); (6) bacterial urinary tract infection; (7) backup of urine into the kidney (hydronephrosis); and (8) kidney failure. Kidney failure is detected by a blood test (BUN and creatinine). Hydronephrosis is detected by X rays (IVP, CAT scan, or MRI) or by renal ultrasound.

WHAT SHOULD THE UROLOGIST DO?

First, the urologist should repeat the history and physical examination.

You're kidding, why does he have to do that? Why does he have to examine my prostate again? It's not a very comfortable thing.

Because the urologist is specially trained, he needs to go into more detail about the nature of your symptoms and the examination. When it comes to examining the prostate for signs of BPH and prostate cancer, the urologist is the expert. He is more experienced at evaluating your particular symptoms and more experienced in making decisions based on his findings. Moreover, he needs to get to know you and you need to get to know him. He needs to know what your priorities or concerns are and how far you want to go with diagnosis and treatment.

What does the urologist do after he has done the history and physical examination?

First, he should sit down and discuss his findings with you and formulate a plan for diagnosis and treatment with which you are comfortable. You should understand what he is saying. You should understand why he has recommended a particular course of action, and you should understand the likely consequences of following his instructions and the consequences of not following them. You should also establish a time frame for the rest of your evaluation and treatment.

At the conclusion of the first visit, he should ask you to complete a preprinted voiding diary and return for a uroflow and postvoid residual urine determination on your next visit. The uroflow measures how forcibly the urine comes out and the postvoid residual urine test determines how well you empty your bladder. Both of these tests are usually done during the same visit. Neither is invasive and neither hurts. The uroflow is obtained by having you urinate into a funnel-shaped receptacle at the bottom of which is an electronic device to measure the rate of urine flow. Postvoid residual urine is estimated by placing an ultrasonic probe on your lower abdomen over the bladder. Postvoid residual urine may also be measured by passing a catheter through the urethra into the bladder, but this is an invasive test that could be a little painful and could cause a urinary tract infection. Whenever possible, I think it is better to measure with ultrasound.

On the basis of this evaluation, the urologist should be able to make a tentative diagnosis and make further recommendations for either attaining a more definite diagnosis or beginning treatment. He should also discuss the advisability of prostate cancer screening, but if he has a suspicion of prostate cancer, he will probably want to order a blood test (PSA) and possibly schedule you for a prostate biopsy. These topics are discussed in detail in the next chapter.

If there is no suspicion of prostate cancer and no signs of infection, he should discuss diagnostic and treatment options with you and then either begin treatment or commence a more sophisticated diagnostic evaluation.

DIAGNOSTIC EVALUATION

The purpose of the diagnostic evaluation is threefold: first, to determine whether your symptoms require further evaluation; second, to determine the specific cause of your symptoms; and third, to determine whether or not the symptoms pose a threat to your health. If the symptoms are not a threat to your health, treatment is entirely elective (you decide whether or not you want to be treated). If the symptoms are a risk to your health, you still decide whether or not you want to be treated, but treatment is strongly recommended. You should be advised of all the risks and benefits and the pros and cons of each treatment, including no treatment at all.

History and Physical Examination

A detailed history and physical examination will be obtained. You might be asked to complete a questionnaire first, and afterward you will have a personal interview with the physician. This helps to pinpoint not only the cause of the symptoms but other conditions that might affect diagnosis or treatment. In addition to the routine physical examination, a detailed examination of the prostate and the nerve supply to the bladder and sphincter is performed. In order to examine the prostate, your physician inserts his gloved, well-lubricated index finger into the rectum. This is called a digital rectal exam (DRE). The technique of DRE is depicted in Figure 2. The examination is uncomfortable, but not painful. The size and consistency of the prostate can be easily determined by examination. This is important because it is the best means for early detection of prostate cancer and also helps to determine the best method of surgical removal of the prostate, should that prove necessary.

Blood Tests

Two blood tests—blood urea nitrogen (BUN) and creatinine—are ordered to check that the kidneys are working normally. These may be combined with a panel of other blood tests.

A third blood test, for PSA (prostatic-specific antigen), may also be ordered. Prostatic-specific antigen is a chemical that is secreted by both the

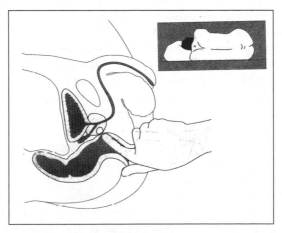

Figure 2. Digital rectal exam (DRE). The doctor inserts a lubricated, gloved finger into the rectum and palpates the size and consistency of the prostate gland. From R. S. Kirby, J. E. Oesterling, & L. J. Denis, *Indispensable Guides to Clinical Practice. Prostate Cancer.* Fast Facts. Clinical Presentation, p. 24, Health Press, Oxford, 1995, with permission.

normal and cancerous prostate gland. It is elevated in patients with large prostate glands and also in patients with prostate cancer. The role of PSA in routine evaluation of prostatism is controversial because there are high false positive and false negative rates. This means that a significant number of men with a high PSA do not have prostate cancer and a significant number of men with prostate cancer have a normal PSA. The whole topic of prostate cancer and screening for prostate cancer is discussed in Chapter 14.

Urine Tests

There are three urine tests that are routinely performed in all men with LUTS: urinalysis, urine culture, and bacterial sensitivities.

Urinalysis

Examination of a fresh specimen of urine is an essential part of the initial examination, which should never be omitted from the initial evaluation unless a recent urinalysis is available. The purpose of the evaluation is to be sure that there are no signs of infection or blood in the urine. In addition, the urinalysis can pick up signs of diabetes and kidney disease. The urinalysis is performed on a "clean catch" or "midstream" sample. A clean catch is obtained in the following fashion: You begin to urinate and once the urine is coming out with a good stream, you catch it in a specimen cup. The reason for obtaining the specimen in this fashion is that the first segment of the urine sample is often contaminated by organisms at the tip of the urethra.

The urinalysis is done in two parts—the "dip stick" test and the microscopic examination. The dip stick is a strip of paper impregnated with a panel of chemicals. Once submerged in the urine, it is removed. Within a minute or so, the chemicals react with different substances in the urine and the paper changes color. The color changes indicate the acidity of the urine (pH) and amounts of red and white blood cells, sugar, protein, and ketones.

After the dip stick test is done, the urine is centrifuged (spun around at very high speed) and then examined under the microscope for red blood cells, white blood cells, and bacteria.

The microscopic examination is very important because the dip stick is often too sensitive. That means it can detect very tiny amounts of blood cells that can be present in normal people. If the dip stick shows blood cells but the microscopic exam does not, the test should be considered normal.

Urine Culture and Sensitivities

If there is a suspicion of urinary tract infection, a urine culture is important to determine whether or not there is infection and to identify the particular kind of bacteria that is causing the infection. Bacterial sensitivities test which antibiotics are effective against the disease-causing bacteria. Many bacteria that cause infection develop resistance to certain antibiotics, which means that antibiotic will not kill the bacteria or cure the infection. It is therefore important to be sure that the antibiotic with which you are being treated is appropriate for the bacteria that is causing your infection.

Cystoscopy

Cystoscopy means literally "looking into the bladder and urethra." It is performed by your urologist, with local anesthesia, by passing a small telescope (cystoscope) through the penis into the bladder. The purpose of cystoscopy is to assess the size of the prostate and to check for other conditions, such as bladder cancer, that might mimic BPH.

I heard that cystoscopy is very painful in men. Why do I have to have it with local anesthesia? Can't you just put me to sleep?

For most men, cystoscopy is uncomfortable, but not terribly painful. There are two types of cystoscopes—flexible ones and rigid ones. Flexible cystoscopes are very similar in size and flexibility to catheters. They are well tolerated by the majority of men, causing little more than a discomfort or slight pain. Rigid ones can be more painful, but even these rarely cause enough pain to warrant more extensive anesthesia. Even when there is pain, it usually lasts only a matter of seconds. Occasionally, though, cystoscopy can be painful enough to require anesthesia. Unless you have a particular fear about the procedure, it is usually best to try it with local anesthesia. If it should prove too painful, your urologist can simply terminate the cystoscopy and reschedule it with anesthesia.

Urodynamic Evaluation

Once infection has been excluded and it has been determined that there is no blood in the urine, urodynamic studies may be done to determine the specific cause of LUTS. In fact, urodynamic testing is the only means by which it is possible to clearly distinguish the different conditions that cause the symptoms of prostatism—a blockage, a weak bladder, or involuntary bladder contractions. Urodynamic studies are performed by passing a small tube (catheter) through the penis into the bladder and another small catheter into the rectum. The bladder is filled through the catheter and the pressure inside of the bladder and rectum is measured during bladder filling and when urinating. The urinary flow rate is also measured and X rays may also be obtained.

Prostate Ultrasound

Prostate ultrasound is another way of "looking" at the prostate. It is performed by passing an ultrasonic probe into the rectum. As the ultrasonic waves are absorbed and reflected by the tissue, an image of the prostate is displayed. If there is a suspicious area that requires biopsy, the ultrasound is a very accurate way of being sure that the biopsy is taken from the right part of the prostate. It is not possible to diagnose prostate cancer from the ultrasound image, nor is prostate cancer screening by ultrasound useful.

TREATMENT OPTIONS

In the great majority of patients, treatment of LUTS is entirely elective. That means that you need treatment only if the symptoms bother you enough. However, there are a few exceptions to this. There are some conditions that require treatment because, without treatment, your health could be impaired. These include the following:

1. Acute urinary retention. This is the total inability to urinate at all, and must be temporarily treated by passing a tube (catheter) into the bladder to release the urine. After that it will be necessary to find the cause and elect a treatment to prevent recurrence and protect against infection and kidney damage. Kidney damage can occur because of backup of pressure through the ureters, and infection can occur because the residual urine in the bladder predisposes to bacterial growth.
2. Damage to the kidneys from the prostate blockage.
3. Severe or recurrent bleeding from the prostate.
4. Severe or recurrent infections due to the prostate.
5. Recurring symptoms from bladder stones.

Under other circumstances, once it has been determined that you do not have cancer of the prostate (as discussed in the next chapter), you need no further treatment than what you think is necessary. For the purposes of this discussion, treatment will be divided into those that are routine and have withstood the test of time and those that are either experimental or quasi-experimental. By quasi-experimental, I refer to new treatments that are FDA approved and being offered to patients, but for which there are no meaningful long-term studies that predict the final beneficial results, complications, or safety. Over the last few years there has been an explosion of new therapies that have received extraordinary attention by the media. In my judgment, most of this is just "hype" and should be viewed in the proper perspective.

Established options include:

1. "Watchful waiting" and behavior modification
2. Medications (alpha blockers)
3. Surgery

New treatments include:

1. Medications (anti-androgens, 5 alpha-reductase inhibitors).
2. Alternate methods of prostatic ablation, including laser, vaporization, thermotherapy, hyperthermia, and cryosurgery.
3. Prostatic stents (hollow tubes that are placed inside the urethra as it goes through the prostate that hold the urethra open and prevent it from being compressed by the growth of prostatic tissue).

Watchful Waiting

If you feel that your symptoms aren't bad enough to warrant treatment, then you don't need treatment (unless you have one of the conditions described above) and watchful waiting is appropriate. Watchful waiting simply means that you return for annual examinations to be sure that there isn't any subtle deterioration in your condition that requires treatment. At these examinations, you should expect to provide an update of your symptoms (a voiding diary is very useful for this) and obtain a urinary flow rate, prostate examination, and blood tests. Further, for some symptoms, behavior modification may be a reasonable option. For example, if one of your symptoms is nocturia (getting up at night to urinate), simply altering your behavior by drinking less after dinner may be effective. If your bladder doesn't hold enough urine, you can learn behavioral techniques to increase its capacity.

Medications

The only medications of *proven* effectiveness for patients with prostate symptoms are the alpha blockers, drugs that relax the muscular tissue in the wall of the prostate. These medications were first developed to treat hypertension (high blood pressure). The most commonly used agents are doxazosin (Cardura) and terazocin (Hytrin), but many more are currently under clinical investigation.

The principal side effects of these medications are related to their effect on blood pressure, namely lightheadedness, dizziness, and even fainting spells. Some patients develop fatigue or headaches. Side effects are not common but, if they do occur, it may be necessary to discontinue the medicine. In order to minimize the likelihood of side effects, the medications are taken at night right before you go to sleep. Your doctor will probably advise you to titrate the medicine. This means that you start at a low dose, then gradually increase the amount of medication until the desired effect is achieved (improvement in your symptoms) or you experience side effects. These medications should not affect your ability to engage in sex. Erections and orgasm are not affected at all, but some men may develop retrograde ejaculation. In retrograde ejaculation, the semen goes into the bladder instead of out the tip of the penis. This is not harmful, and you can't usually even feel the difference. The only negative effect is that it may be difficult or even impossible to father children.

Surgery

The surgical procedures that are used to treat BPH are intended to relieve prostatic obstruction. There are three basic surgical techniques:

1. Transurethral prostatectomy (TURP)
2. Transurethral prostatotomy (transurethral incision of prostate, TUIP)
3. Open prostatectomy

The final results of all of these procedures are comparable. However, the recovery period is longest and complication rates are greatest after open prostatectomy, and least after transurethral prostatotomy. The overall success rate for all of these procedures is approximately 80%. The two major complications are bleeding, which occurs in about 5%, and permanent urinary incontinence, which occurs in under 1% of patients. The chances of dying are 0.2%, but most deaths occur in patients over the age of 85 or those in poor general health.

TURP and TUIP

TURP and TUIP are both done without any incisions at all. A surgical instrument (resectoscope) is passed into the urethra through its opening at

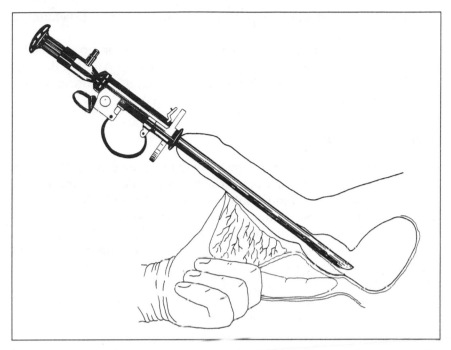

Figure 3. Technique of transurethral resection of the prostate (TURP). A long, telescopelike instrument (called a resectoscope) is passed through the tip of the penis into the urethra. The prostatic tissue is cut out from the inside by removing tiny pieces at a time. From F. Hinman, Jr., *Transurethral Prostatectomy. Benign Prostatic Hypertrophy*, p. 833, Springer-Verlag, New York, 1983, with permission.

the tip of the penis (Figure 3). The resectoscope is passed down the urethra until it is positioned at the prostate. The resectoscope has a cutting instrument at its end (called a loop) and a magnifying telescope so that the surgeon can see what he is doing. Little pieces of tissues are scooped out from the inside of the prostate with the loop. The actual cutting is usually done by the loop, which is heated to very high temperatures using electrical current.

Most people find it difficult to understand how this operation is done. Imagine you pass a straw through the core of an apple. The apple is like the prostate; the straw is like the urethra. Through the straw, you pass the resectoscope. With the loop, first you cut away a piece of the straw from the inside, then little pieces of the apple are removed from the inside until only the skin of the apple is left. Actually, not all of the prostate is removed, since some remains stuck to its capsule, the outer covering of the prostate, like the skin of the apple. Figure 4 depicts the prostate before and after TURP.

In TUIP, no prostatic tissue is removed; rather, one or more radial incisions are made. Visualize looking into the inside of the urethra through the resectoscope (Figure 3). Using a different kind of loop, incisions are made at about 5 and 7 o'clock, opening up the urethra.

Open Prostatectomy

Open prostatectomies are done by making an incision in the lower abdomen, just above the pubic bone. The prostate is identified and shelled out from its capsule. The end result is similar to that of TURP. There are two kinds of open prostatectomy: retropubic and suprapubic prostatectomy. In the suprapubic approach, the bladder is entered through an abdominal incision and the surgeon's finger is passed through the urethra and the prostate is shelled out from the inside, similar to TURP. In the retropubic approach, the same type of abdominal incision is made, but the bladder is not entered. Rather the capsule of the prostate is opened and the prostate tissue removed through the incision.

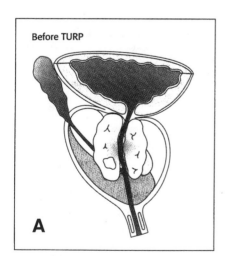 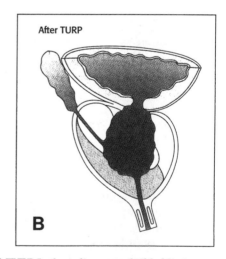

Figure 4. The prostate, before (A) and after (B) TURP. In these diagrams, the bladder is seen above the prostate and the urethra is seen going through the prostate. The urine is dark grey. The duct coming off the left side of the picture is the seminal vesicle.   A. The urethra is narrow as it goes through the prostate.   B. The urethra is greatly widened where the prostate tissue is removed. From R. S. Kirby, J. E. Oesterling, & L. J. Denis, *Indispensable Guides to Clinical Practice. Prostate Cancer. Fast Facts. Clinical Presentation*, p. 23, Health Press, Oxford, 1995, with permission.

Open prostatectomies are only done on prostates that are too large to be safely removed through the transurethral approach, but the particular technique (retropubic or suprapubic) depends on your local anatomy and the preferences and skills of your surgeon. No matter which technique is used, postoperative care is pretty much the same, except that recovery is longer after open prostatectomy. A catheter is generally left in place for a day or two after TURP and TUIP and for 5–10 days after open prostatectomy. The catheter is necessary to drain the urine until you are able to urinate on your own. Immediately after surgery, the urine usually is very bloody, and if you haven't been warned about this, it can be frightening. However, the actual amount of blood loss is usually minimal—it looks much worse than it is. After the catheter is removed, you are given a voiding trial. That means that you wait until your bladder begins to fill with urine from the kidneys, then you try to void when you feel the urge. In the vast majority (well over 90%) of patients urination is easy and complete (but it may still look bloody). If you are not able to urinate or are not comfortable urinating, it may be necessary to pass a catheter again and leave it in place for as long as a few weeks or even a month until healing has occurred.

New Treatments

New treatments are just that. They are not necessarily better or safer; they are just new. In fact, if history is borne out, most new therapies will be either less effective or not as safe as established ones. The new treatments for BPH discussed below are good ideas, usually based on sound hypotheses. Otherwise, they wouldn't be taken seriously and considered new treatments. Nevertheless, only time will tell whether or not they are any good. When considering these new therapies, beware, and be sure to compare them carefully to established therapies.

Alan J. Wein, Professor and Chairman of Urology at the University of Pennsylvania, reminds us of the words of William Heberden, a pioneer of modern medicine: "All new therapies work miracles . . . for a little while." He admonishes us to be careful with all new therapies because many will prove to be either short lived, ineffective, or even harmful. On the other hand, without new treatments, we'd all be stuck in time and no progress would be made.

Medications

5 Alpha-Reductase Inhibitors. These medications block the conversion of the male hormone, testosterone, to dihydrotestosterone. Dihydrotestosterone is the agent that is mainly responsible for growth of the prostate. It is hoped that by blocking this conversion, prostate growth will be slowed or even reversed and that this will reduce symptoms. Finasteride (Proscar) is the only currently available 5 alpha-reductase inhibitor that is FDA approved for treatment of BPH. It has been used for about five years now and, so far, studies have shown that it causes the prostate to shrink by approximately 30% in about two-thirds of male patients. Unfortunately, the overall results have not been very impressive. Those men who seem to derive benefit do so only after taking the medication for about six months.

The medication is well tolerated and side effects are few: 3–5% develop decreased libido and impotence and, in some men, the volume of semen emitted during ejaculation is reduced. These side effects are said to be completely reversible in most cases when the medication is discontinued. Finasteride also causes the PSA level to fall by about 50%. It does not appear to decrease (or increase) the likelihood of developing prostate cancer, but the lowered PSA may make it more difficult to rely on PSA screening for early detection.

Phytotherapy.   Phytotherapy refers to substances used for healing that are derived from plants. The most popular one currently in use is called saw palmetto. At the present time, there are no meaningful scientific studies that document either efficacy or safety of these extracts.

Minimally Invasive Therapies

These are techniques that are intended to mimic the effects of prostate surgery without subjecting the patient to the possibility of serious complications. A number of methods have been designed to destroy the inner part of the prostate and thereby widen the channel and reduce the blockage caused by the enlarged prostate. In all of these techniques, the prostate is heated to temperatures ranging from 41–120°F, causing damage to prostate tissue. The higher the temperature, the greater the damage. At very high temperatures, the prostatic tissue is actually vaporized—it is turned into a gas. Lower temperatures cause death (necrosis) of individual prostate cells. When the cells die, they must eventually be expelled by the body. This is called sloughing—small clumps of necrotic tissue break loose from the prostate and fall into the urethra. Sloughing usually occurs for several weeks after treatment and causes pain as well as frequency and urgency of urination. Unfortunately, in some patients, the sloughed tissue actually causes more blockage. For this reason, when a lot of sloughing is expected, it is often best to leave a catheter in the urethra for several weeks after treatment.

Once necrosis takes place, the final result is the formation of a cavity inside the urethra that widens the channel, reducing the blockage caused by the prostate. The specific techniques for achieving this effect are all either experimental or quasi-experimental, including (1) hyperthermia and thermotherapy, (2) laser ablation, (3) transurethral needle ablation, and (4) high-intensity focused ultrasound. In all of these techniques, there is a variable decrease in symptoms and increase in urinary flow rate.

Because the specific techniques of minimally invasive therapies are being modified so often, it is not possible to give a fair appraisal of the overall results, complications, and safety. If you are interested in any of these treatments, you should discuss the specifics with your doctor. Ask how long the treatment has been available, how long your doctor has been using it, and how many patients he's treated. Ask about side effects and complications. Ask about other treatments that are available and ask why he is recommending this particular one. Ask if other local doctors are using other new techniques not available to your doctor.

Hyperthermia and Thermotherapy.   In hyperthermia, the prostate is heated to 41–45°C. Heating to 45–55°C is called thermotherapy. Hyperthermia and thermotherapy are performed by passing a probe into the rectum or into the urethra close to the prostate. The heating coil may be powered by microwave, circulating water, or radio frequency. It appears that hyperthermia does not heat the prostate to a high enough temperature to cause necrosis and for this reason it is falling out of favor. Heating of the prostate causes the prostatic tissue to become necrotic and over time, the tissue is sloughed off, widening the channel. Some techniques are painful and require anesthesia; others are painless or nearly so.

Treatment consists of one or more heating sessions, each lasting about an hour. In the majority of patients only local anesthesia is necessary but over time the prostate may swell, requiring the temporary use of a catheter. Further, as necrotic tissue continues to be sloughed off, there may be pain and discomfort during urination. During this time, urinary frequency and urgency are common.

Laser Surgery.   Lasers are currently being investigated as another way of destroying prostate tissue. A number of techniques are available. All are painful and therefore require general or regional anesthesia. The laser instrument can be inserted through a cystoscope and operated under direct vision by the surgeon. This is called endoscopic laser ablation of the prostate (ELAP). Another technique, which places the laser instrument directly into the prostate, is called interstitial laser therapy. In the short term, laser therapies appear to be reasonably effective and improve uroflow. However, there have not yet been enough studies to evaluate either long-term efficacy or safety.

Transurethral Needle Ablation (TUNA).   Transurethral needle ablation of the prostate is another method of applying heat to the prostate. Tiny needles are inserted into the prostate and radio frequency energy is applied to heat the prostate to about 120°F. Its safety and efficacy appear to be about the same as the laser techniques.

High Intensity Focused Ultrasound.   In this technique, an ultrasound probe is placed in the rectum and ultrasound waves are transmitted to the prostate to cause it to heat up to temperatures of about 90–100°F. As you might have guessed, its efficacy and safety appear to be about the same as the other techniques.

Prostatic Stents

Another approach to relieving the obstruction caused by the prostate is to simply bypass it with a tube called a prostatic stent. Prostatic stents are basically hollow tubes, made of a wire mesh, that are passed into the prostatic urethra to hold the walls apart, thereby bypassing the blockage. This is basically the same technique that is used in the coronary arteries to treat heart attack victims. These stents may be used on a temporary or permanent basis. However, there have been a number of problems associated with stents and they are not used very often except in patients whose medical health is so poor that other treatments seem too risky. The main problems include formation of clumps of calcium on the mesh (encrustation) and movement of the stent into the bladder or too far into the urethra. This may result in infection, bleeding, and difficulties with urination.

How to Decide on the Best Treatment for You

For most men, treatment of BPH and LUTS is entirely elective. Of course, you must first undergo a diagnostic evaluation, as outlined above, to be sure of the cause of your symptoms and to be sure that treatment is not necessary to protect your health.

OK, I've done that and the doctors said that any treatment is elective. Now what?

First, you should decide how badly your symptoms bother you and whether you think you need any treatment at all. You might notice that you urinate a little more frequently than previously, that the force of your stream is becoming weaker and that you are starting to get up at night to urinate. At first, this may cause concern because you're afraid that it might be the beginning of something more serious. If that's not the case, you may decide to forego any treatment at all and that is fine. However, you should be checked on a yearly basis thereafter, by your doctor, preferably a urologist, to determine whether you will need treatment down the line.

If you feel that your symptoms are bothersome enough now, you should consider the pros and cons of all the treatment options, discuss them with your doctor, and then make your own decision based on his advice. When discussing treatment with your doctor, be specific. Go through the following checklist.

1. How long has the treatment been available?
2. How long has your doctor been using it?
3. How many patients has your doctor treated?
4. What are the side effects and complications?
5. Are other treatments available?
6. Are other local doctors using other new techniques not available to your doctor?
7. Why does your doctor recommend this particular one?

Table 1 summarizes currently available options.

Table 1. Comparison of Treatment Options for BPH and LUTS

Treatment outcome	Watchful waiting	TURP	TUIP	Open prostatectomy	Alpha blockers	Finasteride
Chances of improvement in symptoms	31–50%	75–96%	78–83%	94–99%	59–86%	54–78%
Degree of improvement	?	85%	73%	79%	51%	31%
Chances of 67 y/o man dying within 3 months	0.8%	.53–3.3%	.2–1.5%	.99–5.7%	.8%	.8%
Risk of incontinence	?	.68–1.4%	.06–1.1%	.34–.74%	?	?
Retrograde ejaculation	0%	25–99%	6–55%	36–95%	4–11%	0
Loss of work (days)	1–2	7–21	7–21	21–28	3.5	1.5
Hospital stay (days)	0	1–5	1–3	3–10	0	0

CONCLUSION

Lower urinary tract symptoms in men are one of the most common afflictions of advancing age, but they may also be present in young men as well. Although most commonly attributed to prostate problems, there are many other causes and, for nearly all patients, effective treatment is available. In the majority of patients, treatment is elective, but an accurate diagnosis is important to exclude more serious conditions such as bladder or prostate cancer. In certain instances treatment is important because of the possible ill effects on health if it is not begun. Effective treatment is based on a clear understanding of the basic causes underlying symptoms. In order to diagnose these underlying causes a basic evaluation is necessary.

14

Prostate Cancer

Prostate cancer is the most common malignancy affecting men over the age of 50; 244,000 new cases of prostate cancer were diagnosed in 1996 in the USA alone. Over the course of a lifetime, about one out of three men will develop prostate cancer and about 3% of men will die of prostate cancer. At autopsy, 80% of men dying from all causes have microscopic evidence of prostate cancer; astonishingly, 30% of men dying of accidental deaths in their thirties have microscopic evidence of prostate cancer. Interestingly, prostate cancer differs from most other cancers. Most men who have prostate cancer live out a normal life and don't even know they have it. On the other hand, cancer of the prostate is second only to cancer of the lung as the most common cause of cancer deaths in men. An explanation is in order.

Prostatic cancer has a very variable natural history. Many patients live 15 or 20 or more years with cancer of the prostate, have no symptoms at all, and eventually die of something else; other patients are dead within a year or two of their first symptom. In a sense, you can think of two different kinds of prostate cancer, a more benign kind and a more malignant kind. Even though most men have the benign kind (and live out a normal life and die of something else), because it is so common, there are enough men with the malignant kind to make it the second leading cause of cancer deaths in men. Not all experts agree with what I just told you about prostate cancer. In fact, most experts don't agree with that and certainly, most urologists don't agree with that. Most urologists think that all prostate cancer is bad, and that what I call the malignant kind is just that much worse. They think that if a man has prostate cancer, and it is not treated, he will eventually die of the prostate cancer. They think that early diagnosis and treatment are crucial and that prostate cancer screening is a very important health care issue. They would argue that if a man has prostate cancer and he lives long enough, he will eventually die of prostate cancer unless it is treated. They would argue that my opinion is wrong because prostate cancer is usually diagnosed in old men and they simply die of something else before the prostate cancer can kill them.

The champion of this viewpoint is Patrick Walsh, Professor and Chairman of the Department of Urology at Johns Hopkins Medical School. Dr. Walsh believes that prostate cancer is a lethal disease, that early diagnosis and treatment are essential for cure, and that surgical treatment (radical prostatectomy) offers the best chance of cure. Dr. Walsh has been a pioneer in the surgical treatment of prostate cancer, but until recently, relatively few men with prostate cancer would agree to undergo radical prostatectomy. One of the main obstacles was the fact that after this surgery, nearly all men developed the inability to obtain erections (erectile impotence). About 15 years ago, Dr. Walsh discovered the work of Professor Peter Donker in Leiden. Toward the culmination of a brilliant academic career, Professor Donker, also a urologist, became interested in the nervous supply to the bladder and prostate. In the course of painstaking anatomic dissections, he discovered the exact course of the nerves that are involved with erection as they went past the prostate. When Dr. Walsh learned of Professor Donker's work, he postulated that if these nerves could be preserved, then the most common complication of radical prostate surgery—erectile impotence—might be prevented. With the aid of Professor Donker's anatomic dissections, Dr. Walsh modified the existing surgical technique and devised a way of removing the cancerous prostate without damaging these delicate nerves. His new operation, called nerve sparing radical retropubic prostatectomy, has become a mainstay of prostate cancer treatment. The possibility of maintaining sexual function after radical prostatectomy has led many men to consider potential curative surgery, whereas previously they might have elected other forms of treatment.

PROSTATE CANCER SCREENING

In 1766, Thomas Jefferson, at the tender age of 23, voyaged to Philadelphia to be vaccinated against smallpox. The decision to be vaccinated was not an easy one. Although smallpox was a deadly killer, the vaccine itself could be deadly and it was thought that inoculated persons actually spread the disease. Few doctors would even dare to perform the inoculation for fear of killing the patient. It was not until 1798, 22 years later, that Dr. Edward Jenner reported on the use of cowpox vaccine, a much safer way to be vaccinated against smallpox, and even then, it took another four years before most doctors began to use the vaccine. Nevertheless, Jefferson believed in the vaccine and he lived to be over 80 years of age.

What does Thomas Jefferson's decision to be vaccinated have to do with prostate cancer screening? Did he know something that others of his generation did not know? Was he just smarter? Or was he just plain lucky? In 1766, not many doctors knew very much about smallpox, and in 1998, not many doctors know enough about prostate cancer to advise patients exactly what they ought to do. Just as Thomas Jefferson had to make his own decision about whether or not to get vaccinated against smallpox, you have to make your own decision about whether to get screened for prostate cancer and how you want to be treated if you should develop prostate cancer.

In the majority of men with prostate cancer, the condition shows no symptoms at all for many years (perhaps decades) and the only way it can be detected is by examination of the prostate or a blood test called PSA. Examination of the prostate is done by inserting a gloved, lubricated finger into the rectum and feeling the gland. This is commonly done as part of a routine annual physical exam and is called digital rectal exam, or DRE.

PSA is an abbreviation for prostate-specific antigen, a protein that is secreted by both normal and cancerous prostate tissue. In the bloodstream, some of the PSA is free and some is bound (attached) to proteins. Each can be measured separately and reported as total and free PSA. Just as the prostate grows with advancing age, so does PSA increase with increasing age and prostate size. The relationship between age, prostate size, and PSA level is a complicated one, and many doctors believe that there are age-specific and size-specific normal values of PSA. On average, though, most accept a PSA value of less than 4 nanograms per deciliter (ng/dl) to be normal. For values between 4 and 10 ng/dl, the chances of prostate cancer are about 20% and there is an increasing chance as the PSA rises. However, PSA also rises as the prostate enlarges, so there is no exact way to determine whether or not there is cancer by measuring PSA alone. Recently, it has been suggested that measurement of free PSA in the blood might be a more accurate way of screening for prostate cancer. The lower the ratio of free PSA to total PSA, the greater the chances of prostate cancer. Men with less than 25% free PSA are thought to have the greatest chance of having prostate cancer.

Further, many men have prostate cancer even though the PSA is not elevated. No matter what, though, there is no way of being certain whether or not prostate cancer is present without doing a prostate biopsy.

In the early stages, carcinoma of the prostate is usually not evident at all on examination and can only be detected by prostate cancer screening with PSA. As the disease becomes clinically manifest, it may be suspected because your doctor feels a small hardness or lump on the prostate during rectal examination. During the rectal examination, your doctor inserts his gloved, lubricated finger into the rectum to feel the prostate. It may be done with you lying on your side, knees flexed against your chest (Figure 1), or standing, bent over at the hips with your hands resting on the examination table. The examination, which takes only a matter of seconds, is uncomfortable, but not painful; most men report feeling a pressure sensation as the prostate is felt. In general, whenever your doctor feels an abnormality on examination that is suspicious for prostate cancer, it should be biopsied unless he thinks there might be a prostate infection or some other condition that does not require immediate biopsy. In some instances, your doctor may not be sure that there is in fact a mass in the prostate and he might recommend that you defer the biopsy and be reexamined in several months, or he might recommend a prostatic ultrasound examination to confirm the presence of an abnormality. Delaying the diagnosis by waiting for the results of a reexamination or prostate ultrasound is neither harmful nor dangerous and might avoid any unnecessary biopsies.

About 30% of men with an elevated PSA (> 4 ng/dl) have prostate cancer and when the PSA > 10, about 60% of patients have prostate cancer. If you believe in early detection and treatment of prostate cancer, it makes sense to obtain an annual PSA.

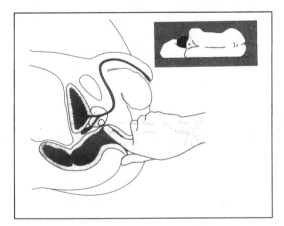

Figure 1. Digital rectal exam (DRE). The doctor inserts a lubricated, gloved finger into the rectum and palpates the size and consistency of the prostate gland. From R. S. Kirby, J. E. Oesterling, & L. J. Denis, *Indispensable Guides to Clinical Practice. Prostate Cancer.* Fast Facts. Clinical Presentation, p. 24, Health Press, Oxford, 1995, with permission.

So, if I want to be sure that I don't die from prostate cancer, I should do annual screening.

No, that's not necessarily true. If you get screened and you have the malignant kind of prostate cancer, even with the best treatment, it could eventually kill you. If you have the more benign form of prostate cancer you might live out a normal life even without any treatment at all. Further, if you live long enough, you'll probably get prostate cancer no matter what you do, but in most instances, you won't even know you have it unless you get screened.

I'm confused. What should I do?

It's a very difficult decision. If you choose to get screened, you'll see your urologist once or twice a year, at which time he will do a rectal examination of the prostate and measure your PSA. If you are an anxious person, you may feel worried, anxious, or nervous each time. (Of course, if you're a worrier, you might also get worried if you haven't gone for an exam.) Eventually, your doctor will probably detect either an abnormality on rectal exam or a rise in the PSA and he'll want to do a prostate biopsy. If it is negative, and he is still suspicious of prostate cancer, he might want to repeat the biopsy. This whole scenario can play out many times until one day when the biopsy comes back positive, you will have to decide how (and whether) to treat it.

What if I don't get screened? What if I do have prostate cancer?

If it's the more benign kind, it probably doesn't make that much of a difference. If it's the more malignant kind, it could kill you. But let me repeat, not all urologists agree with my viewpoint. In fact, only a minority do.

Why don't I just get screened, then. If it's the more benign kind, I'll be OK, and if it's the more malignant kind, I'll get early diagnosis and treatment.

That makes good sense, but right now, it's just not that simple. Treatment of the more malignant kind is not always successful, and there can be significant complications from treatment that alter your lifestyle. Further, we can't even tell with certainty whether you have the more benign or the more malignant kind.

You're not making this a very easy decision for me.

It's not an easy decision, but it is *your* decision. I believe that the decision to undergo prostate cancer screening is the most important decision you make because it more or less dictates what you do next. I've never had a patient who agrees to prostate cancer screening, finds out that he has prostate cancer, and then decides not to treat it. So if you are going to have prostate cancer screening, you should be prepared to make potentially life-altering and even life-threatening decisions about whether you want to be treated, and, if so, how you want to be treated.

I don't understand.

If you'll excuse the analogy, it's kind of like making a decision about whether or not you want to initiate a lawsuit. Imagine that you felt you were wronged by someone—maybe you bought a television set that turned out to be a lemon and you could not get any satisfaction from the dealer. You speak to an attorney and she tells you that you can sue, and if you win, you'll get your money back. But once you start the lawsuit, you can't back out and you've got to pay all the attorney's fees (which she estimates will be $3000). The television only cost $250, so you've got to be pretty sure that you want to do this before you start; there's no way of backing out.

That's the way it is with prostate cancer screening; for most people, once they start, they can't get out. Since, as you get older, prostate cancer is so common, there is a good chance that, if you are screened annually, one day you'll get a biopsy, and eventually be diagnosed with the disease. Then you'll have to decide on treatment. For practical purposes, all potentially curable treatments for prostate cancer have at least a 50% chance of causing impotence or, at best, altering your ability to get erections. All treatments can be complicated by urinary incontinence, excessive bleeding, or other difficulties with urination, and all can cause other complications as well.

So as you can see, prostate cancer screening, diagnosis, and treatment is a very complicated issue; whether or not to undergo screening is a very personal decision. So to a certain extent, your decision about screening will depend on your threshold or tolerance for the possibility of developing impotence or incontinence if you do develop prostate cancer.

What do you mean?

The major complications of treatment for prostate cancer, as I've just mentioned, are impotence and incontinence. If you are already impotent or if you are already incontinent, or the possibility of impotence or incontinence is something that you can accept or deal with, then the decision is not so difficult. But if being impotent or incontinent is something you feel that you could not adjust to, making your decision will be that much more difficult.

I heard that there are far fewer complications with other treatments for prostate cancer like external beam radiation (which does not require surgery) and minor surgical procedures like brachytherapy (insertion of radioactive seeds or pellets directly into the prostate), *high-energy, focused ultrasound, and cryotherapy* (applying extreme cold to the prostate). *What if I choose these treatments?*

There is still a very high likelihood of impotence and there still could be incontinence or other difficulties urinating and the results of these treatments are uncertain.

HOW IS PROSTATE CANCER DIAGNOSED?

Prostate cancer is diagnosed by obtaining a small piece of prostatic tissue and looking at it under the microscope, in other words, a biopsy. The time-honored method of obtaining prostatic tissue for examination under the microscope is the transperineal or transrectal needle biopsy. *Transperineal* and *transrectal* simply refer to where the biopsy needle is passed. A transperineal biopsy is performed by passing the needle through the skin of the perineum (between the scrotum and rectum). A transrectal biopsy is performed by passing the needle through the rectum into the prostate. Either technique is usually performed on an outpatient basis and the only anesthesia usually required is local anesthesia (like the dentist uses). Most of the time the biopsy is done with ultrasound guidance. That means that an ultrasonic probe is placed in the rectum, which shows the prostate and the biopsy needle on a screen. That way the doctor knows exactly from where he is taking the biopsy.

So you use local anesthesia; great, that means it doesn't hurt.

I didn't say it didn't hurt, I said that anesthesia generally isn't required. It does hurt. It just doesn't hurt very much or for very long. Some people are queasy. The thought of a little pain or discomfort makes them very anxious. If you are particularly anxious or frightened, monitored anesthesia care (MAC) might be a good idea. With this method, the biopsy is scheduled with the attendance of an anesthesiologist who can administer anesthesia if it is necessary. Usually an intravenous line is started, and depending on the degree of discomfort that you experience, the anesthesiologist can administer some medications through the intravenous line or, if necessary, give you a general anesthesia and put you to sleep for the examination if the pain is intense enough.

If the biopsy is performed with ultrasound, you'll be lying on your side, sort of in the fetal position. The ultrasound probe is inserted into the rectum and the needle is passed through the probe into the prostate (Figure 2). The doctor checks the position of the needle, then activates the biopsy gun. You hear a "pop," but usually there is no pain.

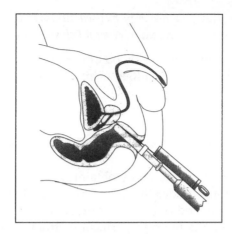

Figure 2. Ultrasound guided prostate biopsy. From R. S. Kirby, J. E. Oesterling, & L. J. Denis, *Indispensable Guides to Clinical Practice. Prostate Cancer.* Fast Facts. Clinical Presentation, p. 24, Health Press, Oxford, 1995, with permission.

A transperineal biopsy is performed with you lying on your back with your legs placed in stirrups so that your hips and knees are flexed. This is called the dorsal lithotomy position. After the penis and rectal area are thoroughly washed with an antibacterial solution, sterile drapes are placed all around the site of the biopsy to prevent infection. The urologist places his index finger in the rectum and feels the abnormality on the prostate. Then, after injecting a local anesthetic, such as Xylocaine, he advances a special needle, called a biopsy needle, directly into the abnormality and through the needle removes a small piece of tissue for biopsy.

No matter which method of biopsy is used, as soon as the examination is over, you can leave. There may be some blood in the urine for several days and there also may be blood mixed with sperm during sexual encounters. Both of these conditions are normal and are no cause for concern. However, should you pass blood clots or have difficulty urinating, you should see your doctor.

No cause for concern? Thanks a lot. I don't need you to tell me that if I see blood clots in my urine or semen and if I can't urinate at all, there's no cause for concern.

Seeing blood in the urine or semen is actually quite common after prostate biopsy and not a sign of a more serious condition. It does not mean that you have cancer and it almost never requires any treatment other than drinking more fluid. However, if you have an excessive amount of bleeding, difficulty urinating, or if you have fever or chills, you need to see your urologist. He should check that you are able to urinate adequately, that you're not leaving too much urine behind, and that you don't have an infection. He will obtain a urinalysis and a culture to make sure that there is no infection and he will examine you. He should repeat the rectal examination and palpate (feel) the bladder. If he is satisfied that you are emptying your bladder alright, he will probably just advise you to drink a lot of fluids. If he is not sure or if you're not emptying, he should do a bladder ultrasound. If he finds a large amount of residual urine, then he'll have to pass a catheter through the penis into the bladder, rinse out the bladder and irrigate the clots and then, depending on the severity of your symptoms, either take the catheter out and have you try to void once again, or leave the catheter in to give the bladder a rest for a few days.

AFTER THE PROSTATE BIOPSY

Okay. So my prostate's been biopsied. Now what?

Now you wait for the results. If the biopsy shows benign prostatic hyperplasia, you don't need any further evaluation or treatment now, but you should make yearly visits to your urologist so he can check the growth of the prostate. If the biopsy does show cancer of the prostate, further evaluation and treatment will depend on a variety of factors that are really beyond the scope of this book.

Beyond the scope of this book! I have cancer and you want me to buy another book? Thanks a lot. I bought this book and I want you to tell me about prostate cancer.

OK, here goes.

As we've already discussed, prostate cancer is very common. The older you are, the greater your chances of having it. At age 80, about three-quarters of all men have at least microscopic evidence of prostate cancer. As compared to many other kinds of cancer, prostate cancer is often relatively slow growing. In many patients it causes no symptoms. In others, however, it is fatal. Treatment depends on a number of factors, including the patient's age, his overall state of health, and the stage and grade of the tumor. The grade of the prostate cancer refers to the appearance of the tumor under the microscope. There are two grading systems, or scores, in common usage. In both systems, the higher the number, the greater the chances that the tumor will spread. The most widely used system is the Gleason score, which is based on how closely the tumor cells resemble the normal glandular architecture of prostatic tissue. This system recognizes five grades, but since prostate cancer may have a different appearance in different parts of the same prostate, the number of the two most common grades are added together. For example, if the cancer cells are grade 1 in one part of the prostate and grade 4 in another, the Gleason score is reported as $1 + 4 = 5$.

The stage of the tumor refers to how far the growth of the tumor has progressed. There are two widely accepted staging systems: the Jewett system and the TMN system. The Jewett system classifies the tumor into four stages, A–D. In Stages A and B, the prostate tumor is confined to the prostate gland. In Stage C, the prostate tumor has grown outside of the prostate itself but is confined to the local tissue around it. In Stage D, the prostate cancer has spread to other organs such as the bone, liver, or lungs. The TMN system is much more elaborate and is depicted in Table 1.

Here're a few examples of how the grading and staging systems work. A Gleason's $2 + 1 = 3$, T2, N0, M0 prostate cancer means that the

Table 1. The TMN Classification of Prostate Cancer

Prostate tumor
T1	=	Incidental (impalpable and not detectable by ultrasonography)
T1a	=	Well-differentiated prostate cancer diagnosed at transurethral resection of the prostate (TURP) involving less than 5% of resected prostate tissue
T1b	=	Any tumor diagnosed at TURP that is less than well differentiated and/or involves more than 5% of resected material
T1c	=	Impalpable prostate cancer diagnosed on transrectal ultrasonography (TRUS); guided biopsy performed because of elevated PSA value
T2	=	Locally confined to the prostate
T3	=	Locally extensive
T4	=	Fixation onto, or invasion of, neighboring organs

Lymph nodes
N0	=	No regional lymph node metastasis
N1	=	Metastasis in single regional lymph node ≤ 2 cm in largest dimension
N2	=	Metastasis in single regional lymph node > 2 cm but ≤ 5 cm
N3	=	Metastasis in regional lymph node > 5 cm in largest dimension

Distant metastasis
M0	=	No distant metastasis
M1	=	Distant metastasis
M1a	=	Metastasis in nonregional lymph nodes
M1b	=	Metastasis in bone
M1c	=	Metastasis in other sites

cancer has a low grade under the microscope (Gleason's grade 3), the cancer is confined to the prostate (T2), and there is neither spread to local lymph nodes (N0) nor distant metastases (M0). This is a very favorable tumor that has an excellent prognosis and is likely to be cured by radical prostatectomy. A Gleason's 4 + 5 = 9, T3, N2, M1b is a tumor with a much worse prognosis, one for which curative therapies are generally not attempted. Gleason's 9 means that the tumor is poorly differentiated and very aggressive under the microscope. T3 means that it has already spread throughout the prostatic capsule into the surrounding tissue, it is in the local lymph nodes (N2), and it has spread to the bone (M1b) as well.

TREATMENT OF PROSTATE CANCER

Treatment of prostate cancer should be individualized according to the specific characteristics of the patient and his tumor. Because prostate cancer is often slow growing, many older patients forego any treatment at all. The reason for this is that if they have no symptoms now, there is a good chance that they will never develop symptoms and they will die of old age or something else before the prostate cancer is even evident. Before treatment decisions can even be made, it is important to determine the stage and grade of the tumor and, particularly, whether or not the cancer has spread (metastasized). The most common sites of spread are to the lymph nodes, bones, liver, and lungs. Obviously, the spread to other organs is life threatening.

The PSA and the grade of the tumor give important clues about the possibility of metastasis. The higher the PSA and the higher the grade, the greater the chance that metastasis has already occurred. As a general rule, if the PSA is less than 10, metastasis is very unlikely. But no matter how high the PSA, there is no certainty of metastasis. To check for metastasis it may be necessary to do further testing such as CAT or bone scans. Further, if you are considering surgical removal of the prostate (radical prostatectomy), it is important to know that the cancer is limited to the prostate itself. To know for sure, it may be necessary to undergo surgery to remove the lymph nodes, which are the most common sites of spread. This is known as lymphadenectomy, or commonly as a "node dissection." This can be done as a separate operation by laparoscopy, or it may be done at the time of prostate surgery. In either case, if there has been spread to the lymph nodes, the radical prostatectomy generally should not be done, because there is no significant benefit to be derived by removing the prostate if the tumor has already spread.

Once it has been determined that the cancer is confined to the prostate there are two main treatment options available—radical prostatectomy and radiation therapy.

Radical Prostatectomy

There are two methods of prostatectomy that are appropriate for prostate cancer—radical retropubic prostatectomy (RRP) and radical perineal prostatectomy (RPP) (radical means that the entire prostate is removed, not just the cancerous part). There are a number of differences between RPP and RRP. RRP is done through a large incision in the abdomen and may have considerably more blood loss and a longer recovery period than RPP. On the other hand, lymph node dissection can be done through the same incision and it is possible to do a "nerve sparing" operation, which reduces the chances of postoperative impotence. RPP is done through a small incision and has less blood loss and a much easier recovery, but does not allow for a lymph node dissection and it makes impotence much more likely. Both of these procedures require great skill and expertise on the part of the surgeon. Not all urologists possess this expertise and even among those that do, some are much better at one technique than the other.

How do I know if my urologist is better at one or the other technique? How do I know which operation to choose?

Ask the urologist. Ask him which operation he is more familiar with and how many of each he does each year. Ask him why he recommends what he does and what are the pros and cons of each. You can check with his staff and you can check his reputation with other doctors that you see or know. In addition, there is a book called *Best Doctors in America*. It lists the best doctors in America, as judged by their peers and their reputations. As one of the "peers" in urology, I've read that book and can personally attest to the competence of nearly every one of the urologists listed. But beware of magazines that list the best doctor in each major metropolitan region. I've read some of those, too. Don't believe everything you read!

Radiotherapy

Radiotherapy is the application of high-energy radioactive waves directly to the prostate. You can think of this as if you were pointing a shotgun at the prostate. The shotgun pellets hit the cancer cells and cause cellular death (necrosis). However, if you miss your target, the pellets will kill whatever other cells are in their path. Further, like a shotgun, it is impossible to hit just one tiny spot; there is always the possibility of some scatter that results in damage to some of the normal tissue surrounding the cancerous tissue. The most important of these tissues are those in the rectum, the intestine, the bladder, and the urinary sphincter. Damage to them can cause many side effects and complications. For this reason, radiation therapy requires a sophisticated calculation of the exact dose of waves to be applied and the waves must be directed or aimed exactly at the cancerous tissue, being careful to spare the normal tissue. This kind of therapy requires considerable expertise on the part of the radiotherapist (radiation oncologist) who plans and supervises the treatment.

There are two basic kinds of radiation treatment—external beam radiotherapy and interstitial radiotherapy, also known as brachytherapy. External beam radiotherapy is administered by an X-ray machine that generates the radiation waves and aims them at the cancerous prostate tissue. Actually, it is the whole prostate and some of the adjacent tissue that receive the radiation, which is usually applied daily for about six weeks. In addition to the prostatic tissue, it is sometimes advisable to radiate the lymph nodes that drain the prostate in attempt to control spread of the tumor cells.

One of the problems with conventional external beam radiation is that the radiation dose affects normal adjacent tissue, which can cause complications such as bowel and bladder injury. To reduce these complications and to enhance the delivery of radiation to the prostate, a new technique has been developed. It is called three-dimensional conformal radiation therapy. Using advanced X-ray techniques, a three-dimensional image of the prostate and surrounding tissue is constructed and the radiation dose is calculated to conform exactly to this image, sparing the surrounding tissue from potentially harmful X rays.

Interstitial radiation, or brachytherapy, is administered through radioactive seeds or pellets that are placed into and around the prostate. About the size of cooked grains of rice, these seeds can be implanted either with long needles passed through the skin into the prostate or with a surgical procedure that exposes the prostate so that the seeds can be directly implanted under vision.

WHAT IF THE TUMOR HAS ALREADY SPREAD?

If the tumor has already spread beyond the prostate at the time of diagnosis and is causing symptoms, such as difficulty urinating or pain, there are many treatments that are of great benefit. In most patients, the tumor is due, at least in part, to the presence of the male hormone testosterone. Accordingly, treatments that reduce or eliminate the production of testosterone are usually very efficacious. There are two ways to reduce testosterone production—by surgical removal of the testicles (orchiectomy) or by the administration of medications that block the production of testosterone. The female hormone estrogen is very effective at reducing testosterone production. However, administration of estrogen to men does post the threat of other complications, particularly heart attacks and blood clots, and for this reason, it is not used very often. Other medications have proven to be just as effective and much safer. The two most common are leuprolide (Leupron) and goserelin (Zoladex). These medications are administered by intramuscular injection given at monthly or even three-month intervals.

CONCLUSION

Prostate cancer is the most common malignancy afflicting men over the age of 50 and it is the second leading cause of cancer deaths in older men. Yet there is considerable controversy about whether or not routine screening should be performed, whether all men diagnosed with prostate cancer should be treated, and even what constitutes optimal treatment. Many men with prostate cancer never have symptoms, live out a normal life, die of something else, and never even knew that they had prostate cancer; others are dead within a few years of diagnosis. Recently, a new blood test, the PSA, has become available for prostate cancer screening. The decision whether or not to undergo screening is a very personal one that depends, in part, on your age, your overall health, and many other factors. Fortunately, there are very many effective therapies for prostate cancer, and unlike many other types of cancer, there are many effective therapies even when the disease has spread (metastasized) to other parts of the body.

15

Bladder Cancer

At age 56, Marie thought that she had just another bladder infection. She had experienced at least one bladder infection every year for the past decade, and this felt no different. She felt burning when she urinated and had marked frequency of urination. She went to her doctor and he checked her urine and told her that she had an infection. She was treated with antibiotics, and after a few days she was much better. The urine test did, indeed, show infection. A month later, though, she still had frequency of urination and a little burning. There were no more signs of infection in her urine test, but she did have microhematuria (blood in the urine as seen under the microscope). Another round of antibiotics made no difference; neither did pain medications. After a month the symptoms were unchanged and there was still blood in the urine. She didn't feel sick; in fact, she felt quite well, but the urinary frequency and slight burning just didn't let up.

Her doctor referred her to a urologist, who did cystoscopy (looking into the bladder) in his office. He saw a little growth in the bladder that looked like a tiny piece of broccoli except that it had a reddish color. He told Marie that she had bladder cancer and that she'd need a small operation to biopsy it and completely remove it. At first she panicked; when people get cancer, they die, she thought. But her urologist told her not to worry. Bladder cancer is common and treatable. Marie had heard *that* before. "Treatable" meant surgery and chemotherapy and hair loss—and then you die. That's what she thought. She was scared.

Marie had the surgery and was home the next day. Her doctor told her that she did, indeed, have bladder cancer, but it was completely removed and she'd be fine. He was right. Ever since, though, Marie goes to the urologist every three months to have a checkup. Each time he does another cystoscopy, and each time he tells her she is fine, but she has to come back in three more months to get another checkup. She's done this for the last five years and twice he found another bladder cancer and twice the cancer was removed. Marie feels fine, she looks fine, and she has no symptoms. The chances are that she'll continue to live a normal life into old age, but she does need a lifetime of surveillance to be sure that the cancer is held in check.

BACKGROUND

Bladder cancer is not uncommon. After prostate cancer, it is the most common urinary tract cancer. In the United States, approximately 50,000 new cases of bladder cancer are diagnosed each year and about 11,000 people die of it. Over the last 15 years, the annual incidence of bladder cancer has increased by nearly a third. It is thought that this is probably due to environmental carcinogens as discussed below. It is three times more common in men than women and is most common in middle and old age. Whites are affected about twice as often as blacks. Fortunately, when caught in its early stages, bladder cancer is usually treatable and curable.

Risk Factors

In addition to advancing age, there are other risk factors for the development of bladder cancer. These include cigarette smoking, occupational risks (exposure to certain chemicals at work), radiation treatment, and long-term indwelling bladder catheters.

Cigarette Smoking

Most authorities now agree that people who smoke cigarettes have as much as a fourfold increase in the incidence of bladder cancer when compared to nonsmokers. In fact, about 50% of bladder cancer in the United States is thought to be caused, in part, by cigarette smoking. It is thought that some of the breakdown products of nicotine, including a group of substances known as nitrosamines and alpha- and beta-naphthylamines, are the causative agents. These substances are known carcinogens, substances that cause cancer in laboratory animals.

Occupational Risks

Bladder cancer was one of the first cancers that was proven to be caused by a carcinogen. It was discovered that people who worked with certain chemicals known as aromatic amines had an extraordinarily high risk of developing bladder cancer. Further, the longer they worked with this chemical, the greater their chances of developing bladder cancer, and the closer they worked with it, the greater their chances. Subsequently, other chemicals were proven to cause bladder cancer. The most well known of these include benzidene, beta-naphthylamine, and 4-amino-biphenyl. Occupations at risk for developing bladder cancer are listed in Table 1.

Long-Term Indwelling Bladder Catheters

People who are treated with an indwelling bladder catheter on a continuing basis have as much as a tenfold increased chance of developing squamous cell bladder cancer. The longer it stays in, the greater the chances of developing the cancer.

Other Factors

Cyclophosphamide (Cytoxan), a very effective chemotherapy medicine used for many different types of cancer, actually increases the risk of bladder cancer ninefold. It is believed that one of the breakdown products of Cytoxan, called acrolein, is the responsible carcinogen. Further, patients using Cytoxan tend to get more aggressive kinds of bladder cancer, so it is particularly important that these patients be followed closely. If they develop hematuria, a full evaluation should be done to insure early diagnosis and treatment.

Table 1. Occupations at Risk for Bladder Cancer

Plastics workers
Leather workers
Hairdressers
Metalworkers
Painters
Tailors
Carpenters
Food processors
Petroleum workers
Shoe-repair workers
Plumbers
Photographers

Artificial sweeteners have also been suspected to cause bladder cancer, but there really isn't enough evidence in humans to implicate them. In very large doses, artificial sweeteners do cause bladder tumors in laboratory animals, but almost all authorities agree that those dosages are so large that they have no meaning for human bladder cancer. I do not believe that the theoretical risk of bladder cancer from artificial sweeteners is sufficient to be of concern.

HOW TO MAKE THE DIAGNOSIS

In the great majority of patients, bladder cancer is detected because of blood in the urine. The blood may be visible only under the microscope (in which case it's called microscopic hematuria), or the urine itself may be quite bloody, just as if you'd cut yourself. For this reason, any blood in the urine, whether it's visible to the naked eye or only through microscopic evaluation, should be thoroughly investigated by a urologist. In the majority of patients bladder cancer is diagnosed during an evaluation for hematuria.

Whenever there is blood in the urine, the first step in diagnosis is to expand on the patient's history.

Overwhelmingly, the most common cause of blood in the urine is urinary tract infection, particularly in women; next are kidney stones. Both infection and kidney stones can be suspected by the history. Patients with infection complain of the usual symptoms of urinary frequency, urgency, pain during urination, and if the kidneys are infected, fever, chills, nausea, vomiting, and back pain. Kidney stones usually are characterized by severe pain in the back or abdomen associated with blood in the urine. Often there may be frequency and urgency of urination as well. Most people who experience severe bouts of kidney stones say that it is the worst pain that they have ever experienced (including childbirth).

No matter what the history though, the first step in diagnosis is to obtain a urinalysis and a urine culture. If, in addition to blood in the urine, there are also many white blood cells (pus cells) and you have the characteristic symptoms of infection, that is the likeliest cause. The presence or absence of infection is confirmed by the urine culture, which will reveal the offending bacteria. In young people and in children, though, there are sometimes infections with viral organisms that do not grow out on culture, and rarely, as discussed in the chapter on infections (Chapter 10), there are other kinds of infections that do not show up on routine culture.

I guess that means that if I have blood in my urine and I have an infection, then I can rest easy that I don't have cancer?

In the overwhelming majority of patients that's true. However, in older women and men, there is a possibility that you could have both a urinary tract infection and cancer. For that reason it is important to have a complete evaluation, as discussed below, before getting a clean bill of health. If you have a urinary tract infection and also hematuria, once the infection is cured you should get periodic urinalyses over the next few months to be sure there isn't recurrent hematuria without infection. Further, if you are at high risk it's a good idea to get urinary cytologies as well, or if you have persistent symptoms in the absence of infection, further evaluation is also necessary.

Once infection is excluded as the cause of the hematuria, it is important to determine the site of the bleeding and to be sure that the kidneys are functioning normally. Kidney function tests, BUN (blood urinary nitrogen) and creatinine, should be determined. If these are normal, an X ray of the kidney (intravenous pyelogram or CAT scan) should be obtained. Intravenous pyelogram (IVP) is done by injecting a radiographic contrast material (a dye) into your arm, which is concentrated by the kidney. The IVP, which colors the urine white on the X ray, shows the outline of the kidneys and the urine as it goes from the kidneys through the ureter into the bladder. If there are kidney tumors or stones or cysts, they are usually readily diagnosed from the IVP.

CAT scan stands for computerized axial tomography. This kind of X ray is a much more detailed view of the kidney and the entire abdomen than an IVP. The choice between IVP and CAT scan will be made by your doctor. Sometimes it's necessary to get both examinations.

One note of caution, though. Rarely, the IVP radiographic contrast material can cause allergic or toxic reactions and kidney damage. If you have an allergic history or a specific allergy to contrast material you should discuss this with your physician and the radiologist doing the X ray. Further, if you have certain other risk factors, including diabetes, dehydration, or impaired renal function (as measured by the creatinine), you may require other treatment before the X ray is done or it may be advisable to do other kinds of imaging that do not require the contrast material.

After the upper urinary tract (kidney and ureter) has been evaluated by X ray, the next step is cystoscopy. Cystoscopy, discussed in more detail in Chapter 4, is visual examination of the bladder with a small telescope. The entire bladder and urethra may be visualized, and if the bladder or urethra is the source of the bleeding, the cause is usually apparent. If a bladder tumor is suspected, a biopsy will be necessary in order to obtain a definite diagnosis. Most bladder tumors have a characteristic, unmistakable appearance. In its most classic form, the bladder cancer resembles a small cauliflower or broccoli, except that it is reddish in color. Sometimes the lesion has a more reddish moundlike appearance and sometimes there are just some flat areas of redness. If any of these lesions are present, it is necessary to biopsy the bladder. In the case of the flat, red lesions, it is usually possible to obtain a biopsy under local anesthesia, or if the other kinds of lesions are small enough they too may be biopsied with local anesthesia. Whenever possible, it is best to completely remove the lesion. If this can be accomplished, diagnosis and treatment are performed in the same session. No matter what, after the tissue is removed, it is examined under the microscope and a definitive diagnosis is made.

TYPES OF BLADDER CANCER

Upon microscopic examination of bladder cells, several different types of bladder cancer can be detected: transitional cell cancer, squamous cell cancer, and adenocarcinoma. These are all primarily bladder cancers—those that arise from the cells in the bladder itself. Very rarely, there may be secondary bladder cancers. These are cancers that have spread to the bladder from other organs. The most common sites from which cancer may spread to the bladder are the adjacent female organs such as the uterus, cervix, or vagina.

The most common type of primary bladder cancer is transitional cell carcinoma (TCC), which accounts for about 90% of all bladder cancers. Next is squamous cell carcinoma, which is seen in 5–10%, and, finally, adenocarcinoma, which is seen in about 2%. Transitional cell cancers are most often associated with cigarette smoking and the occupational hazards depicted in Table 1. Squamous cell cancers are often seen in people who have had chronic bladder inflammation due to infection, stones, or long-term use of catheters. In addition, people with infections due to *Schistosoma haematobium,* a parasite acquired from bathing in infected waters, have a higher risk of developing squamous cell carcinoma. Another name for a schistosomiasis infection is bilharziasis. It is almost unheard of in the United States, but common in certain countries, such as Egypt, where squamous cell carcinoma accounts for about 60% of all bladder cancers. Adenocarcinoma is also most often seen in certain groups of people who are at particularly high risk, which include (1) people who have had tuberculosis of the bladder, (2) people who were born with a rare congenital abnormality called bladder extrophy, and (3) people who were born with another congenital abnormality called patent urachus.

TUMOR STAGE AND GRADE

As for prostate cancer, it is important to determine the stage and grade of the tumor. Grade refers to the microscopic appearance of the tumor and stage refers to how far the tumor has progressed. In general, the higher the grade and the higher the stage, the worse the cancer. Grade is usually reported on a scale of 1–3.

A simple way of looking at bladder cancer is by dividing it into superficial bladder cancer and invasive bladder cancer, depending on whether or not the tumor has invaded the lamina propria, a thin membrane that separates the mucosa of the bladder from the muscle layer. Superficial bladder tumors, which have not penetrated the muscle layer, have a much better prognosis and are usually treated by surgically removing the tumor and a bit of surrounding tissue or by intravesical chemotherapy (putting medicines directly into the bladder with a catheter). Invasive tumors are usually treated by surgical removal of the entire bladder.

Superficial transitional cell carcinoma bladder tumors are further subdivided into papillary tumors and carcinoma in-situ. Papillary tumors, like the one that Marie had, look like reddish pieces of broccoli; carcinoma in-situ usually has the appearance of a reddish flat spot on the bladder wall.

For tumor stage, there are two systems in use: the Jewett system and the TMN system. The Jewett system recognizes four stages, A–D. Stage A refers to a superficial cancer that has not penetrated the lamina propria. Stage B refers to cancer that has invaded the lamina propria and has penetrated the muscle of the bladder wall. B1 refers to superficial muscle invasion and B2 to deeper invasion into the muscle. In Stage C, the tumor has spread through the wall of the bladder, but not into the lymph nodes or other organs of the body (it has not metastasized). In Stage D, the tumor has metastisized to either lymph nodes or other organs.

The TMN staging system refers to the depth of tumor growth (T), involvement of lymph nodes (N), and extent of metastases (M). Tis refers to carcinoma in-situ and Ta refers to a papillary carcinoma that has not invaded the lamina propria. T2 means that the tumor has invaded the superficial layer of muscle, and in T3a, the deeper portions of the bladder wall

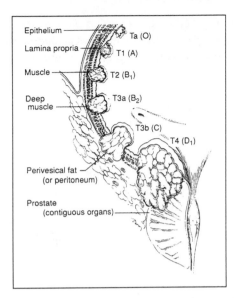

Figure 1. Comparison of the Jewett and TMN systems. This diagram shows the right half of a bladder as it would appear at different stages of bladder cancer. The TMN stages Tis to T4 are shown next to the comparable Jewett stage, listed as letters in parentheses. From P. R. Carrol, E. A. Tanagho, J. W. McAninch, Appleton & Lange, *Smith's General Urology*, 13th edition, Norwalk, 1992, with permission.

are invaded, but the tumor has not penetrated the bladder wall. In stage T3, the tumor has pierced the wall of the bladder, and in stage T4, adjacent organs such as the prostate (in men) or uterus (in women) are invaded. N0 means that all regional lymph nodes are negative for tumor. A single lymph node with cancer that is less than 2 cm in size is deemed N1. If a single lymph node is 2–5 cm in size, it is staged N2, and N3 means that there is one or more lymph nodes greater than 5 cm in size. The staging system is illustrated in Figure 1. For example, a superficial cancer that has not spread to either lymph nodes or other organs might be classified as Ta, N0, M0, whereas an invasive tumor that has spread to the bladder wall and a lymph node, but has not metastasized, would be staged as T2, N1, M0.

TREATMENT OF BLADDER CANCER

Treatment is largely determined by stage and grade. Unlike prostate cancer, there is not too much controversy about how to treat bladder cancer. When considering treatment, two factors need to be considered—

tumor recurrence and tumor progression. Recurrence refers to the tendency of cancer to reappear, even when it has been completely removed by surgery. Tumor progression refers to the tendency of the tumor to become more advanced, either by growing deeper into the tissues or by spreading to other parts of the body (metastasis). Tumor recurrence is very common in patients with bladder cancer; up to 80% will have a recurrence within five years. For those with superficial tumors, the recurrences are easily treated, and the great majority of patients with superficial bladder cancer live out normal lives and die of something else. Because of the tendency for bladder cancer to recur, however, it is essential that after the initial treatment, careful follow-up visits are scheduled every three months. Between visits urinary cytologies should be done on urine specimens. At each visit, a cystoscopy should be performed and, once a year, a kidney X ray (intravenous pyelogram, or IVP) should be done.

There are three methods of treatment for bladder cancer—surgical treatment, chemotherapy, and radiation treatment. Initial treatment always begins with surgery because that is how the diagnosis is made—by transurethral resection and biopsy of the bladder tumor (TURBT). TURBT is done by using a specialized kind of cystoscope called a resectoscope. The resectoscope is passed into the bladder through the urethra and with a cutting electrocautery loop the bladder cancer is completely removed whenever possible. Once the results of the biopsy are known, further treatment depends on the stage and grade.

Treatment of Superficial Bladder Cancer

There are two kinds of superficial transitional cell carcinoma (TCC)—papillary TCC and carcinoma in-situ (CIS).

Papillary TCC

For patients with superficial papillary TCC (stage A in the Jewett system or Ta in the TMN system), treatment is always surgical and the intent is to completely remove all cancer cells by TURBT. If there are multiple tumors, as there often are, they are all removed during the same surgery. If the tumor is small, superficial, and of low grade, no further treatment is necessary provided that the tumor has been completely removed. Of course, careful surveillance with periodic follow-up as outlined above should be maintained. If the tumor is of high grade (grade 3), multiple, or associated with a known carcinogen, most authorities recommend that intravesical chemotherapy be administered. Intravesical chemotherapy is administered by first passing a catheter through the urethra into the bladder and emptying out the urine, after which a few ounces of the chemotherapy agent is instilled into the bladder through the catheter. The catheter is removed and you are asked to turn from side to side and to try to retain the chemotherapy agent for as long as possible, preferably for one to two hours. There are a few different kinds of intravesical chemotherapy agents. Some have rather long names—triethylenethiophosphoramide (Thiotepa), Bacille Calmette-Guerin (BCG), Mitomycin C, and doxorubicin (Adriamycin). For prevention of recurrences of superficial TCC, they all work equally well, but BCG and Thiotepa are much less expensive.

Carcinoma In-Situ (CIS)

The characteristic appearance of carcinoma in-situ is a flat reddish spot on the surface of the interior of the bladder (the mucosa). Sometimes it has a velvety appearance. In-situ cancer means that there are cancer cells present, but they have not penetrated through the lamina propria. Initial treatment is the same as for papillary TCC—by TURBT—but if the tumor is extensive, it may not be possible to resect all of it. In these instances the remaining tumor should be coagulated. Coagulation means that the tissue is heated with the resectoscope until the individual cells die.

Once the diagnosis of carcinoma in-situ has been made, surveillance is the same as for the other kind of superficial bladder cancer, but in addition, intravesical chemotherapy is a necessary part of therapy. For CIS, BCG is the best chemotherapeutic agent.

Treatment of Invasive Bladder Cancer

Once the bladder cancer has become invasive (Jewett stages B–D; TMN stages T1–T4), treatment decisions are more complicated. Of utmost importance is surgical removal of all of the cancer and prevention of spread. The surest way of accomplishing this is to remove the entire bladder along with its surrounding tissues and the lymph nodes that drain the bladder. This is a major operation called radical cystectomy and pelvic lymph node dissection. Once the bladder is removed, a new method for handling urine storage and emptying must be found. There are two basic ways of accomplishing this—by constructing a urinary reservoir or a urinary conduit. The time-honored method is the urinary conduit, but for many reasons, it has fallen out of favor and in fact has a number of disadvantages. In my judgment it should only be used when a reservoir is unacceptable. In a conduit, after the bladder is removed, a segment of intestine is separated from the rest of the intestines and connected to the ureters on one end and to the skin of the abdomen on the other end. Urine then drains from the kidneys through the ureters into the conduit and out through a stoma (an opening in the abdomen). The stoma is fashioned in such a way that the urine is collected and then stored in a urinary drainage bag on the abdomen (Figure 2).

There are many problems with urinary conduits. First and foremost is the need for an external urinary drainage bag. From a purely psychosocial standpoint this has obvious drawbacks. Further, over the long term (more than 10 years) there may be significant complications, including kidney stones, recurring infections, and blockage to the ureters. There is the pos-

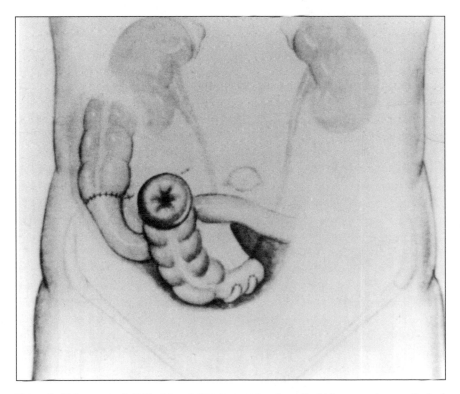

Figure 2. Urinary conduit (ileal loop). The two ureters from the kidney are shown attached to a short segment of intestine (the conduit). The other end of the intestine comes out to the skin. The puckered opening is called a stoma. Urine drains from the kidneys through ureters, into the conduit, and out the stoma into a drainage bag on the skin (not pictured), where it is stored.

sibility of bowel obstruction or the need for further surgeries to revise either the stoma or the conduit itself.

A urinary reservoir is fashioned by utilizing the intestine in a similar way to a conduit, except rather than simply transporting urine from the ureters to the external drainage bag, in a reservoir the intestine is made to resemble a bladder and store urine internally. A stoma is created in the skin as well, but the stoma has a valve mechanism built in so that there is not leakage of urine. Rather, three to four times a day a catheter is passed through the stoma into the reservoir and the urine empties through self-catheterization. With a reservoir, there is still a chance of having the kinds of complications that are seen with a conduit, but the chances are much reduced with the reservoir. Figure 3 depicts a urinary reservoir.

These surgeries sound gruesome. Either I'll have to wear a bag on my side with urine draining into it for the rest of my life or I'll have to catheterize myself for the rest of my life. Aren't there any other ways of handling this?

Radical cystectomy is considered, by urologists, to be *the most conservative* treatment. Patients consider it to be radical treatment, and it certainly is, but it offers the best chance of cure.

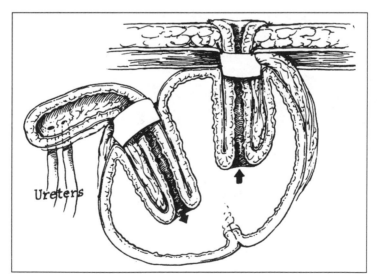

Figure 3. Urinary reservoir. This urinary reservoir is constructed from a segment of intestine that is disconnected from the rest of the intestine and fashioned into the shape of a sphere. The ureters are connected to one end of the reservoir and the other end is brought out to the skin where it is fashioned so that it will serve as a one-way valve. Urine is stored in the reservoir and periodically emptied by intermittent self-catheterization.

Depending on the stage and grade of the tumor, there are a number of other possibilities. Further, if you think that the treatment seems worse than the disease, you'll probably want to consider other treatment options, even if the chances of cure aren't as high. For patients with fairly low grade (grade 1 or 2), localized tumors (Jewett Stage A or B1 or TMN stage T2, N0, M0), many urologists recommend only TURBT followed by intravesical chemotherapy and careful surveillance as outlined above. If the tumor is high grade (grade 3) but localized (Jewett Stage A, B1, or B2 or TMN stage T1, T2, or T3a), it may be possible to remove only part of the bladder (partial cystectomy). Alternatively, some patients might consider surgery and systemic chemotherapy or radiation treatment. I personally do not recommend radiation treatment for patients with bladder cancer because I think the complications are too great. Radiation causes the bladder to become scarred and its blood supply becomes impaired. The net result is a small-capacity bladder that may cause marked urinary frequency and urgency of urination, pain, and bleeding. Further, if the radiation damage is more severe, the bladder wall can stiffen (low bladder compliance). This results in a high pressure inside of the bladder and may cause kidney problems or incontinence.

CONCLUSION

Bladder cancer is the second most common kind of urinary tract cancer. It is usually detected because of blood in the urine. This underscores the importance of obtaining a full evaluation by a urologist whenever there is bleeding in the urinary tract. There are a number of risk factors for developing bladder cancer. These include cigarette smoking and occupational exposure to certain chemicals and toxins. Fortunately, when diagnosed early, most bladder cancers are treatable and you can live out a normal life. However, unlike many other types of cancer, bladder cancer has a great tendency to recur without spreading to other organs. For this reason, careful surveillance is necessary. Even if the cancer recurs many times in the bladder, it can usually be removed with a simple operation through the cystoscope.

16

(Sphincter) Incontinence in Men

INTRODUCTION

Sphincteric incontinence is the involuntary loss of urine due to malfunction of the urinary sphincter. It's like a leaky faucet. In women, sphincteric incontinence is common; in men, it's uncommon. That's because the sphincter in men is a much more complicated structure than in women. In almost every way, women are more complicated than men, but not when it comes to the anatomy and function of the sphincter. If you are a man and you have sphincteric incontinence, the chances are that you've had a prostate operation or that you have a neurologic disorder like spina bifida.

The urinary sphincter is a specialized structure that lies in the wall of the urethra whose function in both sexes is to maintain urinary control. In men, though, the sphincter serves an additional function; it is also a genital sphincter, which means that during sex, when ejaculation occurs and sperm are ejected into the urethra, the sphincter closes. This prevents sperm from going backward into the bladder and insures that the sperm go out the tip of the penis.

Normally, the urinary sphincter is kept closed, due in large part to contraction of the smooth (involuntary) and striated (voluntary) muscles inside and around the urethral wall. During urination these muscles relax and open, allowing urine to pass through. Of course, if the muscles have become damaged or weakened, they do not stay tightly closed and incontinence can occur. The sphincter is actually composed of a number of different elements, not just muscle. Other components of the urethral wall, including collagen and elastin, provide the architectural framework for the sphincter, like the frame of a house. In addition, the inner lining of the urethra (mucosa) secretes a mucus layer that acts like an additional seal,

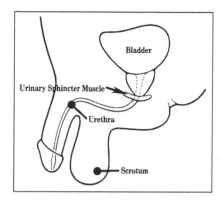

Figure 1. Overall view of urinary sphincter in men. Courtesy of American Medical Systems.

similar to a rubber gasket on a garden hose. In women, this whole arrangement is rather simple. In men, because of the presence of the prostate, the anatomy and function of the urethra are much more complicated (Figure 2).

The junction between the urethra and the bladder is called the bladder neck. Its wall is composed mostly of smooth muscle that is arranged in both a circular and longitudinal pattern around the urethra. The smooth muscle of the urethra is called the internal sphincter. It begins at the bladder neck and is intermingled with the tissue of the prostate. Further, the prostate adds considerable bulk to the sphincter. Consequently, the internal sphincter in men has considerably more strength than in women.

The ejaculatory ducts pass through the prostate and empty into the urethra. Ejaculation, which occurs during the sex act, is the forceful expulsion of sperm, mixed with prostatic secretions, through the ejaculatory ducts, into the urethra, and then out the tip of the penis. There is striated muscle in the wall of the urethra, located mostly just past the prostate and there is striated muscle outside the urethra called the periurethral striated muscle. Together, these muscles constitute the external urethral sphincter, which is much less important than the internal sphincter. If the internal sphincter has been badly damaged, incontinence occurs even if the external sphincter works normally. The main function of the external sphincter is to allow you to suddenly interrupt the stream if you are in the middle of urinating or to hold back once you get a strong urge. If your internal sphincter has been damaged and you have severe incontinence, the chances are that you are still able to momentarily prevent incontinence by contracting your external sphincter. However, since it is a voluntary (striated) muscle, it fatigues easily (after only 10–15 seconds or so) and once that happens the urinary loss continues.

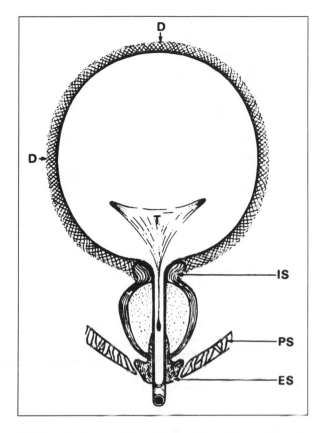

Figure 2. Detailed view of urinary sphincter in men. The urinary sphincter in men is largely in the wall of the prostate, which is wrapped around the urethra. The junction between the urethra and the bladder is called the bladder neck. Its wall is composed mostly of smooth muscle arranged in both a circular and longitudinal pattern around the urethra. The smooth muscle of the urethra is called the internal sphincter. It begins at the bladder neck and is intermingled with the tissue of the prostate. Further, the prostate adds considerable bulk to the sphincter. There is striated muscle in the wall of the urethra, called the external sphincter, which is located just beyond the prostate. There is also striated muscle outside the urethra called the periurethral striated muscle. D, detrusor muscle; IS, internal sphincter muscle; PS, periurethral striated muscle; ES, external urethral sphincter. From J. Gosling, "The Structure of the Bladder Neck and Urethra in Relation to Function," *Urologic Clinics of North America,* 6:31, 1979, with permission.

In women, because the sphincter is naturally much weaker than in men, incontinence is much more common. It occurs, in part, as a consequence of repeated stretching and damage to the nerves and muscles of the sphincter that occur during pregnancy and childbirth, and in part to the effects of gravity, which tend to make the vaginal muscles sag and weaken. Incontinence is so common in women that many consider it a normal part of aging. In men, sphincteric incontinence is rare. It is never a consequence of aging or sphincter muscle weakness; rather, it occurs almost exclusively when the sphincter is damaged by prostatic surgery or radiation treatment for cancer of the prostate. Much less commonly, it may complicate surgery for benign prostatic conditions. It may also occur after radical cancer surgery of the rectum and in certain neurologic conditions. Neurologic causes include spina bifida (myelodysplasia), injuries to the lower spine, and ruptured (herniated) intervertebral discs. There are also a few very rare degenerative neurologic diseases, collectively known as multisystem atrophy, that can cause sphincteric incontinence and, finally, there may be injury to the blood supply of the spinal cord after surgery on the aorta, which results in a condition known as anterior cord syndrome.

POSTPROSTATECTOMY INCONTINENCE (PPI)

The most common cause of incontinence in men is radical prostate surgery for cancer. Radical prostatectomy is complete removal of the prostate, which is performed only for prostate cancer. Incontinence that occurs after radical prostatectomy is called postprostatectomy incontinence (PPI). The prostate itself contains much smooth muscle and contributes to overall sphincteric function. It is no surprise, then, that when the prostate is removed, part of the sphincter is removed with it. This is unavoidable and after prostate surgery, continence depends on the sphincter muscles remaining in the wall of the urethra after the prostate has been removed.

There are two factors that conspire to cause PPI—the skill of the surgeon and the extent to which the prostate cancer itself has involved the sphincter. All things being equal, highly skilled and experienced surgeons have many less complications and much less incontinence than less skilled or less experienced surgeons. However, very often, all things are not equal. More experienced surgeons are more often referred more complicated or more advanced patients. It is possible that, in those circumstances, the complication rate and incontinence rate of the experienced surgeon are even higher than those of the less experienced surgeons. But that is because of the complexity and advanced disease of the patient. Thus, you can't just compare complication rates when choosing a surgeon; it's more complicated than that.

When sphincteric incontinence occurs as a consequence of prostate surgery, there is a very good likelihood that, over the course of time, the sphincter will heal itself and incontinence will no longer be a problem. Unfortunately, this healing process may take an extended period of time, sometimes a year or more from surgery, and in 1–30% of patients, incontinence persists and becomes a frustrating clinical problem.

After radical prostatectomy, most men develop some degree of incontinence, at least for a few days or weeks, but, in the majority, normal urination returns within a matter of weeks or months. However, when incontinence persists, it is impossible to predict whether or not it will subside spontaneously. Thus, conservative treatment should be instituted for as long as necessary until the condition either heals or it becomes obvious that no further improvement is taking place. For practical purposes, it is unwise to consider invasive or surgical treatment until 9–12 months have elapsed since the onset of the urinary incontinence. Thus, treatment is divided into two stages—a "temporizing" stage and a definitive stage.

Postprostatectomy incontinence may also complicate operations for benign prostatic diseases such as benign prostatic hyperplasia, but this is quite uncommon, afflicting less than 1% of such patients (provided that patients were selected properly).

What does that mean, "provided that patients were selected properly?"

Deciding on the advisability of prostate surgery can be very difficult. Some patients undergoing surgery are at much higher risk than others for developing PPI.

I don't understand. Why would a doctor recommend prostate surgery and why would I agree to it if I'm going to be incontinent afterwards?

It's not that simple. Most people who are at high risk for developing incontinence after prostate surgery do just fine and are never incontinent; it's just that their chances for developing it are higher. For example, if you're a healthy 55-year-old man undergoing TURP (transurethral prostatectomy), an operation done through a cystoscope that removes only part of the prostate, the chance of your developing PPI is probably no more than 1 in 1000; if you're 85 years old, the chances of developing PPI are about 1 in 20. If you have Parkinson's disease, the chances are probably 1 in 4 that you'll be incontinent afterwards. If you have very mild symptoms, you probably would not even consider surgery with those kinds of odds. On the other hand, if you can barely urinate at all and spend all day worrying about urination or if you are already incontinent, it may well be worth the chance.

Fortunately, for the majority of patients with incontinence after prostate surgery, the symptoms subside within several months. When symptoms do persist, however, diagnosis and treatment pose a considerable challenge to patient and doctor alike. Postprostatectomy incontinence can be caused by sphincter malfunction, involuntary bladder contractions, or urethral obstruction. Involuntary bladder contractions may be caused by many different conditions—urinary tract infection, a blockage in the urethra, bladder stones, cancer of the bladder, or retained stitches or other foreign bodies accidentally left over from surgery. Further, there may be a neurologic condition, unrelated to the surgery, that causes the involuntary bladder contractions. Sometimes men develop such conditions after surgery, but more often they were present beforehand, but not diagnosed because they were so subtle.

Another bladder condition that can cause incontinence is low bladder compliance. Bladder compliance refers to the volume/pressure relationship of the bladder. It is a measure of bladder stiffness calculated by measuring the change in bladder volume over the change in bladder pressure. Normally as the bladder fills with urine, bladder pressure remains very low despite very large changes in bladder volume. This results in high bladder compliance, which is normal. In other words, in patients with low bladder compliance, the bladder pressure rises considerably with incremental increases in bladder volume. This rise in pressure may overcome the resistance offered by the urethra and cause incontinence. On the other hand, if the sphincter is strong or there is a blockage in the urethra, the high bladder pressure is transmitted back to the kidneys and ureters where it can cause considerable damage. Low bladder compliance is usually due to longstanding urethral obstruction or a rare neurologic condition such as spina bifida.

From a diagnostic standpoint, most people who complain of a constant, dribbling, gravitational or stress-induced incontinence have sphincteric incontinence, and most who complain of urinary frequency, urgency, and urge incontinence have involuntary bladder contractions. However, there may be considerable overlap between these two conditions and both may coexist in the same patient. Another cause of postprostatectomy incontinence is urinary retention with overflow incontinence. In this condition, there is either a severe urethral blockage or a weak bladder, which results in incomplete bladder emptying. What urination there is, is really just an overflow because the main problem is the retention of urine in the bladder. The symptoms—marked urinary frequency and a weak, interrupted, or dribbling stream—can be confused with urinary tract infection or a primary problem of incontinence.

A complete list of the possible causes of postprostatectomy incontinence is shown in Table 1.

Table 1. Common Causes of Postprostatectomy Urinary Incontinence

1. Sphincteric damage
2. Involuntary bladder contractions
3. Urinary tract infection
4. Urethral stricture or scar
5. Cancer of the bladder
6. Bladder stones
7. Retained sutures (stitches)
8. Low bladder compliance
9. Neurologic conditions (stroke, Parkinson's disease, multiple sclerosis)
10. Urinary retention with overflow

INITIAL DIAGNOSTIC EVALUATION AND TREATMENT

After almost all prostate surgeries, a urethral catheter is left in place for a few days to a few weeks depending on the type and nature of surgery. In the first few weeks after removal of the catheter many patients develop temporary urinary frequency, urgency, and urge incontinence. Although the symptoms usually subside spontaneously within a few months, even at this early stage, it is important that your doctor exclude two treatable conditions—urinary tract infection and urinary retention. Infection is diagnosed by urinalysis and urine culture. If you do have an infection, it should be treated with culture-specific antibiotics (antibiotics that have been shown to be effective against the particular bacteria that are causing your infection). Urinary retention means that either you cannot urinate at all or, even though you urinate a bit, you are not emptying your bladder and are leaving a large amount of urine behind. You may not have any symptoms of urinary retention other than frequency of urination and incontinence, but your doctor should be able to diagnose it easily by palpating (feeling) a distended bladder in your lower abdomen. He can confirm the diagnosis by checking with an ultrasound or by passing a catheter through the urethra into the bladder and measuring the amount of residual urine after you void. If you do have urinary retention, it should be treated with an indwelling catheter until the surgery has healed (usually a few weeks). If you still can't urinate well after that, it will be necessary to do some more tests to determine whether the cause is a urethral blockage or a weak bladder. In order to make this distinction, two further tests are necessary—cystoscopy (a visual examination of the bladder) and urodynamic evaluation. Urodynamics refers to one or more of a series of tests that are designed to diagnose the cause of your bladder symptoms.

To perform these tests a small catheter is passed through your urethra and into the bladder and another into the rectum. The bladder is filled with fluid and you will be asked to try to urinate. On the basis of this test, it is possible to determine whether there is a blockage or a weak bladder. If urodynamic study shows a blockage, treatment should be directed by the underlying etiology. The usual causes include a stricture, or scar, or residual prostatic tissue causing obstruction. If a scar is the problem, the only treatment is surgery to cut the scar, but if there is a blockage by the prostate, it is possible that medications will be effective.

If the problem is a weak bladder or a bladder that does not contract at all, self intermittent catheterization (SIC) is the treatment of choice. SIC is done in the following way. Each time you feel the urge to urinate, you try to do so. Whether or not you are successful, you pass a small catheter (a hollow tube) through the urethra into the bladder and empty the remaining urine. For most men, after a period of time, the residual urine will become less and less as the bladder regains its strength, and eventually, the SIC can be discontinued. For some men though, this might be a permanent way to manage the problem.

When urinary retention is not the cause of the urinary incontinence— and it usually is not—for the ensuing weeks to months after surgery management will be very difficult and frustrating for both physician and patient alike. Since the majority of men recover fully, the goals of therapy are to "manage" the incontinence until the symptoms subside. Once more significant conditions such as bladder cancer and urethral blockage have been excluded, you may be treated empirically (by trial and error) based on the presumed underlying etiology. If you have urge incontinence, behavior modification (a bladder-retraining process) or medications to stop involuntary bladder contractions (anticholinergics or tricyclic antidepressants) may be tried. Common anticholinergics include oxybutynin (Ditropan), propantheline (ProBanthine) and hyoscyamine (Levsin). The most commonly used tricyclic is imipramine (Tofranil).

Sphincteric incontinence may be treated with medications that contain alpha-adrenergic agonists such as phenylpropanolamine or pseudoephedrine. These medications—usually found in nonprescription cold remedies—stimulate the vessels in your nose to contract—stop you from sniffling. They also make the smooth muscle of your sphincter and can help with incontinence. If you want to try these kinds of medicines, just read the labels of your cold medicines, make sure that they have either phenylpropanolamine or pseudoephedrine, and take then as if you had a cold. The use of these medications is logical; it certainly makes sense that they should work. But more often than not, they do not work very well.

Further, you should use them with extreme caution if you have hypertension (high blood pressure) because these medications can, and usually do, elevate blood pressure even further. If you have hypertension, you must discuss this treatment with your doctor. Biofeedback may also be tried either alone or in combination with medical treatment.

All combined, these therapies are only occasionally very effective, and at this stage, many patients prefer to use absorbent pads, which are changed as frequently as necessary to keep them comfortable. However, if absorbent pads are unsatisfactory it may be necessary to resort to a condom catheter, penile clamp, or failing that, an indwelling catheter.

SUBSEQUENT EVALUATION AND TREATMENT

Most men will be symptom free by one to two months after prostate surgery, but if you are still incontinent after a few months, it's a good idea to have an evaluation by your doctor.

For mild and moderate degrees of incontinence one of innumerable commercially available absorbent pads may be all that is necessary. If you choose this treatment, it is a good idea to try out a number of different kinds until you find one that best meets your needs. Some men are able to get by with just a thin minipad; others require adult diapers. Alternatively, you might try a penile clamp, a device, usually made of plastic and sponge rubber, that is placed around the base of the penis and tightened just enough so that urinary leakage doesn't occur. Obviously, you have to exercise great care to be sure that you don't put the clamp on so tightly that it damages your penis.

I can assure you that I'd never do that!

While this is rarely a problem in men with normal sensation, if your sensation is diminished, for example, if you have some nerve damage from diabetes, stroke, or multiple sclerosis, you actually could cause damage and not even feel it. All you need to do is periodically check your penis to be sure that there is no swelling or redness. If this does occur, you should simply remove the clamp and leave it off until the swelling and redness subside.

Another form of treatment that you might prefer is a condom catheter. A condom catheter is a sheathlike device that is placed around the penis and secured there with either adhesive or a strap. The other end of the sheath is connected to a small tube that leads to a drainage bag that may be strapped to the leg. Like the penile clamps, it is possible to put a condom catheter on too tightly and damage the penis and, accordingly, you should exercise the same precautions.

The least desirable alternative is the use of an indwelling bladder catheter. Also known as a Foley catheter, it is a plastic tube that is inserted through the penis into the bladder and retained in place by an inflatable balloon at the end of the catheter. Urine drains from the bladder through the catheter into a leg bag, in a similar fashion to the condom catheter. You might find the indwelling catheter preferable to the condom catheter because it is much more secure, and, believe it or not, it is usually quite comfortable. Most of the time, you won't even be conscious of it being there. However, of all the forms of treatment, the indwelling catheter poses the greatest risk to your health. The chances of a serious kidney infection are much greater with a Foley catheter than with the other forms of treatment and there is a possibility that you will develop a urethral stricture, a circumferential scar in the urethra that causes a blockage and can make subsequent treatment of incontinence much more difficult. Further, the catheter itself can become blocked and cause severe pain and infection. For practical purposes, the longer the catheter is used, the greater the chances that you'll develop one of these complications.

If you do choose to use an indwelling catheter, there are a number of precautions you can take to minimize the likelihood of complications. First, you should change the catheter frequently, no less often than every two or three weeks. Blockage of the catheter, manifest by the absence of urine flow for more than an hour or so, is a medical emergency that requires your immediate attention. The first thing you should do is check to be sure that the tubing from the drainage bag is not simply twisted; if it is, when you straighten it out, urine should start to flow immediately. If the tubing is not twisted, the next thing you should do is to irrigate the catheter. This means that you will take a large syringe, fill it with water or an irrigating solution of saline (salt water), and squirt it through the end of the catheter, after disconnecting it from the drainage bag. If this doesn't clear the blockage, it's best if you just change the catheter. I think that it is very important that you learn to do these things so that you can be as independent as possible and not have to rely on family members, nurses, doctors, or worst of all, emergency rooms.

Another form of treatment that you might want to consider is the injection of substances around the urethra that are meant to compress it and thereby improve incontinence. Currently, the most widely used agent is bovine collagen, that is, collagen derived from cows. It's only been available since 1993, so there is little information on the long-term results of this procedure, but it has already been shown to be quite safe and it can be done under local anesthesia in your doctor's office. After injection, collagen is broken down in the body after about 12 weeks, but as part of the breakdown process, new collagen is laid down. The original collagen is completely gone from your body within about one to one and a half years. The procedure has so far been reasonably effective in women with sphincteric incontinence, but the success rate in men is not nearly as good. Only about a third of men have a good response, and this is with multiple injections given over a period of months or years. It is also expensive. On the other hand, there is little to be lost in trying it and some patients have had excellent results for as long as several years. There is a small chance that you could be allergic to collagen, so if you are considering it, you'll need to be skin tested first.

If you are allergic to collagen, and want to try a periurethral injection, it is possible to use autologous fat—that is, your own fat, removed by liposuction from your abdomen. This causes little discomfort and is done in the office under local anesthesia. Overall, its success rate is not even as good as that of collagen.

Because of the relatively low success rate of the currently available injections, a number of other substances are currently being investigated as a replacement for collagen. These include silicone particles, Teflon, and human cartilage.

DEFINITIVE TREATMENT OF SPHINCTERIC INCONTINENCE IN MEN

Currently, the only effective treatment that has stood the test of time for men with sphincteric incontinence is implantation of an artificial urinary sphincter (sphincter prosthesis). There is only one commercially available sphincter prosthesis, that made by American Medical Systems. The sphincter prosthesis, made of a plasticlike material called silastic, consists of three parts: the sphincter cuff, a pump, and a reservoir (Figure 3). The sphincter cuff goes around the urethra and substitutes for the damaged sphincter. The cuff is inflated to compress the urethra so urine may not escape involuntarily. The pressure in the cuff is maintained by a pressure-regulating balloon that is placed in the abdominal cavity during the implantation surgery. A pump is placed in the scrotum so that the cuff may be deflated and the sphincter opened in order to urinate. All three parts are connected by tubing. There are no external parts.

The operation takes about two hours for an experienced surgeon to complete and can be done with general or regional anesthesia. The hospi-

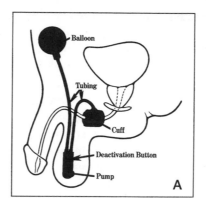

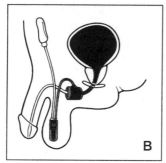
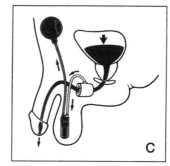

Figure 3. A. Artificial urinary sphincter (sphincter prosthesis). The prosthesis consists of three parts—a cuff that goes around the urethra, a pump that goes in the scrotum, and a reservoir that goes in the abdomen.   B. During normal activities, the cuff is filled with fluid, compressing the urethra and acting like a sphincter.   C. When you want to urinate, you squeeze the control assembly, which empties the cuff, forcing the fluid into the reservoir. The arrows show the direction of fluid transfer into the reservoir. After you are finished voiding, the cuff automatically fills up again after about three minutes. Courtesy of American Medical Systems.

tal stay is a day or two and recovery is four to six weeks. The procedure is usually performed through three very small incisions. One is just underneath your scrotum, another is in the scrotum itself, and the third is in your lower abdomen. In most men, in order to prevent complications, the sphincter is left in the "deactivated state" for four to six weeks after surgery. In this position, the sphincter cuff is in the open position and incontinence is the same or sometimes even worse than it was before the surgery. After the four- to six-week period is up, your doctor will activate the device by squeezing the control mechanism in the scrotum. Until the sphincter is activated, it is necessary to use appropriate aids to deal with the incontinence.

There are three potential complications of major consequence—erosion of the prosthesis, infection, or a mechanical failure. Erosion of the device through the skin of the scrotum or the penis occurs very infrequently, unless there is an accompanying infection. The symptoms of erosion are usually pain in the penis or scrotum and redness and tenderness over the area. After a number of days, the skin over the prosthesis begins to blanch and eventually part of the prosthesis may be seen through the skin. This sounds terribly gruesome, frightening, and painful, but in fact, there is generally no pain at all. Treatment consists of the administration of antibiotics and removal of that portion of the prosthesis. If the wound is clean and no infection is present, it is possible to remove the part of the prosthesis that has extruded and replace it with a new one. However, in most instances it is not advisable to do this, but rather to wait and replace the prosthesis in a second operation, because the risk of infection may seem too great.

It is very unlikely that your prosthesis will become infected; it is a very uncommon complication that is more prevalent in diabetics and in men who are undergoing repeat surgery to the same area. The most common symptom of infection is pain over part of the prosthesis, particularly when you are squeezing the control assembly. Less commonly, there may be fever, redness, and tenderness over the prosthesis. When infection of the prosthesis is suspected, your doctor will prescribe antibiotics; if the infection doesn't respond, the most conservative treatment is to remove the entire prosthesis surgically. After a suitable waiting period of usually no less than two or three months, a new prosthesis may be implanted.

Mechanical failures of the prosthesis occur in about 10% of men over the course of time. These complications include kinking of the tubing, leaks of the connectors of the cuff itself, and malfunctions of the control mechanism. Once a malfunction has been identified, it usually requires a minor operation to replace or fix the malfunctioning part.

CONCLUSION

Sphincteric incontinence in men is uncommon. It is almost always the result of surgery or radiation for prostate cancer, but can also occur after surgery for noncancerous prostate conditions and in certain neurologic conditions like spina bifida. Most of the time, when incontinence occurs after prostate surgery, it subsides within a matter of weeks or months, but occasionally takes a year or more. Treatment is difficult during this stage, but effective methods are available to manage the incontinence until it subsides. For persistent incontinence there are a few treatment options, but the only one that has a good long-term cure rate is surgical implantation of an artificial urinary sphincter (sphincter prosthesis).

17

Neurogenic Bladder

Claire is a 38-year-old freelance writer. She is a quadriplegic, which means that all four of her limbs are paralyzed. She does have partial use of her hands, though, and can type on a computer, one key stroke at a time. For this purpose, she uses a long pencillike device that fits into a special brace that was custom made for her hand. Eighteen years ago, in her senior year of college, she was involved in an auto accident that broke her neck. After two years of intensive therapy, she went back to school and got her bachelor's degree. Last year she won a prestigious literary prize. Hers is a courageous story, but there are lots of quadriplegics who face and overcome similar obstacles.

At first Claire had a terrible time coping with the day-to-day problems that she faced. With the help of a medical assistant, it took her over two hours to get up and out of bed in the morning and another hour to get ready for sleep at night. After about a year, she finally settled into a routine and began slowly to acclimate to her new way of life. By then she could drive a car (a specially equipped van), brush her teeth, and feed herself. She had an electric wheelchair and could take a course at a local college. She needed her assistant only to help her get up in the morning, shower and dress, and get into bed at night. But she couldn't control her urination and had to use a catheter that drained urine into a bag that was strapped to her leg. Sometimes she urinated around the catheter and wet her clothes. She was fearful of the possibility of wetting herself and she worried about the repeated kidney infections that she was experiencing. She felt that her bladder management was keeping her a "patient" and preventing her from leading a more normal life. Incontinence was the only problem that she experienced during her work hours that she couldn't handle by herself. It was the only thing keeping her from being truly independent.

In 1991, Claire learned of a new operation that was being done for quadriplegic women with incontinence, an operation that would free her from the worry of incontinence and repeated infections. The operation involved connecting the bladder to an opening in the belly button called a stoma. Urine could be stored in the bladder until it was full, then emptied by passing a catheter through the stoma. The stoma was constructed in such a way that it acted as a one-way valve and didn't leak urine.

Now you might not think that a quadriplegic would be able to manage all that in her wheelchair—adjusting her clothes to expose the stoma, taking out the catheter and passing it into the stoma, emptying the urine into the toilet or a receptacle without spilling it, and putting the catheter away. I didn't think a quadriplegic could do that either, but with an incredible sense of self-determination many quadriplegics can do just that.

A good friend and colleague of mine, Edward McGuire, Professor and Chairman of Urology at the University of Texas in Houston, was, as far as I know, the first surgeon to do such an operation on a quadriplegic woman. He knew that his patient would be able to catheterize herself and become independent and he was right.

Now, thanks to that operation and her own perseverance, Claire is able to work and lead an independent and productive life.

NORMAL AND ABNORMAL URINARY CONTROL MECHANISMS

Normally, you control your own bladder. It fills painlessly and unconsciously. It tells you when it's time to urinate, but *you* tell it when and where. The bladder is normally under the control of the nervous system. That means that your bladder and sphincter are connected to your brain by nerves. The brain sends messages to the bladder and sphincter, telling them when to relax and when to contract. The bladder and sphincter send messages back to the brain telling it when they want to contract and relax. For example, imagine you are talking to a friend and you get a sudden urge to urinate. Your bladder sends a message to your brain that it is time to urinate, but your brain immediately sends back the message "not now." Normally when that happens, you can delay urination until a socially acceptable time.

If the nerves to the bladder are not working properly, bladder control is lost. This condition is called a neurogenic bladder. Before we discuss neurogenic bladder further, it is necessary to have a better understanding of how the bladder nerves work and what can go wrong. Normally, as your bladder fills with urine, the bladder nerves send messages to the spinal cord that the bladder is filling. As the bladder continues to fill, the nerves send more and more messages back to the spinal cord, but until a critical threshold is reached, these messages never get through to the brain. However, once that threshold is reached, the message is sent to your brain that it is time to urinate. When your brain gets that signal, it must make a choice. If it's not a good time to urinate, it sends down a signal, a chemical message, telling the sphincter to contract and the bladder to relax. In this way, you temporarily postpone urination. If it is OK to urinate, your brain says OK and sends back a chemical message that causes the sphincter to relax and the bladder to contract. The urethra opens and normal urination ensues. This orderly sequence of events—sphincter relaxation, bladder contraction, opening of the urethra, and the onset of urinary flow—is called the micturition reflex (Figure 1). The micturition reflex, as simple as it seems, is a finely tuned neurologic event that requires coordination and integration from many parts of the nervous system. When there is damage to any part of the nervous system involved in the micturition reflex, urination is affected. The particular way that micturition is affected depends on what part of the nervous system is damaged.

The micturition reflex is coordinated and integrated in a part of the brain called the pons, in a region called the pontine micturition center (PMC) (Figure 2). The PMC is the central control mechanism; it receives and sends messages to other parts of the brain and spinal cord. For example, the frontal cortex is a region of the brain concerned with awareness of bladder events and voluntary control over the sphincter muscle. So when a critical threshold is reached during bladder filling, the bladder nerves send messages through the spinal cord to the PMC informing it that the bladder is filling. This, in turn, is relayed to the frontal cortex. The frontal cortex sends a message back down to the PMC telling it whether or not it's OK to urinate. These messages are then relayed to another micturition center located in the lower spinal cord called the sacral micturition center (SMC). From there, depending on the message, either a micturition reflex is begun and urination occurs or the sphincter contracts, bladder contraction is inhibited, and urination is postponed.

When the neural connections between the PMC and the SMC are intact, when urination occurs, it is the result of a coordinated micturition reflex. However, if the connections between other parts of the brain and the PMC are lost, the person may lose control of urination. In this case, incontinence is the result of an involuntary micturition reflex. Imagine that you are driving your car and the brakes fail. You can still steer and accelerate and everything works normally, except you can't stop. That's what hap-

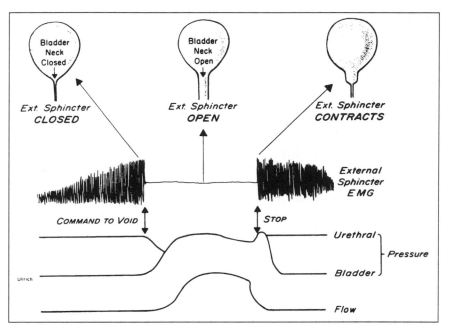

Figure 1. Micturition reflex. Normally, as the bladder fills with urine from the kidneys, the pressure in the bladder remains low and fairly constant. The pressure in the urethra remains greater than the pressure in the bladder, and the bladder neck and external urethral sphincter remain closed so that leakage of urine does not occur. The electrical activity of the sphincter muscle, known as the electromyographic (EMG) activity, gradually increases as the bladder fills. Urination begins with a sudden and complete relaxation of the external sphincter, evident as a cessation of EMG activity and a fall in the pressure in the urethra (marked on this tracing as Command to Void). The urethra opens widely as the sphincter relaxes. Almost immediately, the bladder begins to contract, seen as a rise in bladder pressure, and urine begins to flow, evident on the urine flow tracing. This orderly sequence of events—relaxation of the sphincter, contraction of the bladder, and opening of the urethra—is termed the micturition reflex. Urination ceases with contraction of the muscles of the external urethral sphincter (marked at the arrow indicating Stop). The contracting sphincter cuts off the urinary stream and this causes a momentary rise in urethral and bladder pressure. Within seconds, the bladder stops contracting. From J. G. Blaivas, "Pathophysiology of Lower Urinary Tract Dysfunction," *Urologic Clinics of North America*, 12:215, 1985, with permission.

pens when there is a neurologic lesion between the PMC and other parts of the brain. Everything works normally; it's just that you can't stop urination once it wants to start. This commonly occurs in conditions such as stroke (cerebrovascular accident), Parkinson's disease, multiple sclerosis, and brain tumor.

When the connections between the PMC and SMC are disrupted, the result is usually a condition called detrusor–external sphincter dyssynergia (dee-troo-sor/sfinkter/diss-sin-urgia) (DESD). *Detrusor* is the medical

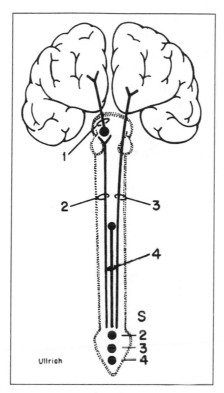

Figure 2. Neurologic control of the bladder and sphincter. The micturition reflex is coordinated by the pontine micturition center (PMC), located in the pons, a part of the brain just above the spinal cord. The PMC is marked by a black circle at pathway 1. The PMC sends and receives messages from the sacral micturition center (SMC), which is located in the sacral portion of the spinal cord in sacral segments (S2–4). The connection between the PMC and SMC is pathway 2 in this diagram. When neurologic disease interrupts this pathway, the micturition reflex becomes uncoordinated, a condition known as detrusor sphincter dyssynergia. Voluntary control of micturition is accomplished by connections between many different parts of the brain and the PMC (pathway 1). When these pathways are damaged, voluntary control of micturition is lost and the person develops urinary incontinence. The SMC and the thoracolumbar center contain the nerves that make the bladder and sphincter contract and relax under the control of the PMC (pathway 4). Another set of connections, between a part of the brain called the frontal cortex and the SMC (pathway 3) is necessary for a person to contract his or her sphincter to stop the urinary stream or to prevent urination. From J. G. Blaivas, "Pathophysiology of Lower Urinary Tract Dysfunction," *Urologic Clinics of North America,* 12:215, 1985, with permission.

term for the muscle of the bladder and dyssynergia means that the action of two muscles oppose one another. In DESD, the coordination between the bladder and sphincter is lost and the sphincter contracts during bladder contraction instead of relaxing. In effect, there is a blockage to the flow of urine by the person's own sphincter. However, the bladder contraction eventually overcomes the sphincter contraction and incontinence occurs. People with DESD are both obstructed (by their own sphincter contraction) and incontinent (because of the involuntary detrusor contraction). The obstruction in these people is very serious and, without treatment, usually causes serious kidney damage that can lead to kidney failure and even death. Common causes of DESD include spinal cord injury, multiple sclerosis, and spina bifida (myelodysplasia).

In the SMC are located the nerves that regulate bladder and sphincter contraction, called the pelvic nerve and the pudendal nerve. These nerves also carry the impulses for bladder and sphincter sensation (Figure 3). The pelvic nerve is a parasympathetic nerve. It sends its messages with a chemical neurotransmitter called acetylcholine. Parasympathetic nerves supply (innervate) organs like the heart and intestine over which there is

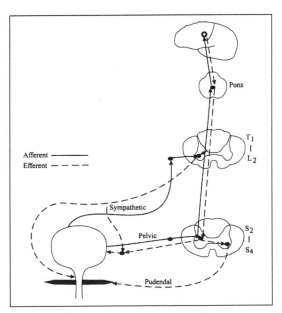

Figure 3. Sacral and thoracolumbar nervous supply to the bladder and sphincter. There are three sets of nerves that supply the bladder and sphincter—the sympathetic nerve, the parasympathetic nerve (pelvic nerve) and the somatic nerve (pudendal nerve). The sympathetic nerve arises in the thoracolumbar part of the spinal cord (T1–L2). Stimulation of this nerve makes the sphincter contract and the bladder relax. The pelvic nerve comes from the sacral micturition center (SMC) in the sacral part of the spinal cord (S2–S4). The pelvic nerve makes the bladder contract. The pudendal nerve also comes from the SMC and makes the sphincter contract. From M. B. Chancellor, & J. B. Blaivas, *Genitourinary Complications in Neurologic Disease, Practical Neuro-Urology*, Butterworth-Heinemann, Boston, 1995, with permission.

no voluntary control. The pudendal nerve is a somatic nerve. Somatic nerves supply tissues over which you have voluntary control, like the muscles in your arm. It also uses acetylcholine as its neurotransmitter. A third nerve, the hypogastric nerve, carries sympathetic fibers to the bladder and sphincter. This nerve arises above the SMC in a part of the spinal cord called the thoracolumbar region. The sympathetic nerve does not feel sorry for the bladder and sphincter; rather, it sends impulses mediated by a neurotransmitter called norepinephrine, which makes the bladder relax and the sphincter contract, thus promoting continence and preventing micturition. Like the parasympathetic nerves, there is normally no voluntary control over the muscles innervated by the sympathetic nervous system.

When the SMC is damaged, there is a variable effect on the micturition reflex depending on which of the nerves are injured. If the pelvic nerve is injured, the bladder can no longer contract, and the person is unable to urinate at all and will require a catheter to empty the bladder. If the hypogastric nerve or pudendal nerve is injured, the sphincter might not work properly and sphincteric incontinence occurs. If both the pelvic and hypogastric or pudendal nerves are injured a paradoxical situation arises. There is urinary retention (because the bladder cannot contract) and incontinence (because the sphincter doesn't work). Common causes of SMC disruption include spinal cord injury, multiple sclerosis, diabetes mellitus, ruptured (herniated) intervertebral spinal discs, spina bifida, and gunshot wounds to the lower spine.

TREATMENT OVERVIEW

Although the ultimate goal of therapy is the restoration of normal voiding, this is usually not possible unless the neurologic condition is cured or remits, or if the symptoms are caused by a coincidental urologic condition such as blockage by the prostate gland in a man or stress incontinence in a woman. When you are trying to decide about treatment, your own feelings about your symptoms—their effects on your day-to-day life and their consequences, particularly incontinence—must always be weighed against the potential risks to your general health imposed by the treatments themselves. For example, if you are a woman with mild incontinence due to involuntary bladder contractions, you may prefer to manage your symptoms with incontinence pads (which pose no threat to your health) rather than with an indwelling bladder catheter (which can cause repeated urinary infections and kidney stones).

Table 1. Classification of Voiding Dysfunction

Storage problems (insufficient capacity or incontinence)
    A.   Bladder overactivity
        1. Detrusor hyperreflexia (the bladder contracts involuntarily)
        2. Low bladder compliance (the bladder wall becomes too stiff)
    B.   Sphincter weakness
Emptying problems
    A.   Weak or absent bladder contractions
    B.   Urethral blockage
Storage and emptying problems
    A.   Detrusor–external sphincter dyssynergia (uncoordinated urination)
    B.   Urethral blockage and bladder overactivity
    C.   Weak or absent bladder contractions and sphincteric weakness
    D.   Low bladder compliance and sphincter weakness

After you've had an evaluation of your symptoms, the cause can be classified as filling/storage abnormalities, emptying abnormalities, or a combination of the two. Treatment should be directed at the underlying abnormality that is responsible for the symptom. Table 1 depicts this classification system in regard to neurogenic bladder.

Treatment is dependent on the cause of the symptoms. For bladder overactivity, treatment is usually directed at abolishing the involuntary bladder contractions. Medications are generally tried first, including anticholinergics such as oxybutynin (Ditropan), propantheline (ProBanthine), dicyclomine (Bentyl), flavoxate (Urispas), and hyoscyamine (Cystospaz, Levsin). Tricyclic antidepressants, such as imipramine (Tofranil), are tried if the anticholinergics fail. They may be used alone or in combination with an anticholinergic. In people with neurogenic bladder, these medications are often so effective that the person is unable to urinate at all. For most people, though, this is a blessing in disguise because they become totally dry and can manage themselves with intermittent catheterization.

If the medications are ineffective, and symptoms are bad enough, surgery can be considered. The most effective operation is augmentation cystoplasty. This is a major surgical procedure in which the bladder is enlarged using a piece of your own intestine (see Chapter 20). The purpose of this operation is to greatly increase the capacity of the bladder (increase the volume of urine that the bladder can hold before you urinate) and to prevent the bladder from contracting involuntarily. The success rate of augmentation cystoplasty is over 90%, but, just as it is with anticholinergic medications, you will be unable to urinate naturally afterward and you'll have to do intermittent self-catheterization. If you are a man, you should be able to catheterize yourself without difficulty. You'll be able to learn in less than a half hour; it will be painless, clean, and no big deal. Most women can also do SIC without difficulty, but if your neurologic condition causes spasticity of your legs, it may be very difficult for you to catheterize yourself while you are in your wheelchair.

Whether you are a man or a woman, if you cannot catheterize yourself through your urethra, other surgeries are possible and very effective. You can undergo an operation like Claire had. She underwent an augmentation cystoplasty, where a piece of her intestine was used to connect the bladder to the abdomen at the belly button, creating a stoma, an opening in the abdomen that connects to the urinary tract (Figure 4). The stoma may be a continent one or an incontinent one. If you choose a continent stoma, you'll have to catheterize it three to five times a day. An incontinent stoma requires you to use an appliance that lies on your abdomen, attached to the stoma. Urine drains into the appliance, which is usually connected to a leg bag where the urine is stored. You'll have to empty the leg bag periodically (two or three times) throughout the day.

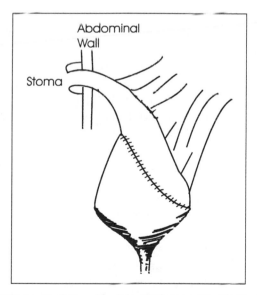

Figure 4. Augmentation cystoplasty with abdominal stoma. The bladder is enlarged with a piece of intestine and an opening (stoma) is made in the skin of the abdominal wall, usually near the belly button. The bladder can be emptied by passing a catheter through the stoma or a bag may be worn on the abdomen to collect the urine. From M. B. Chancellor & J. G. Blaivas, *Genitourinary Complications* in *Neurologic Disease, Practical Neuro-Urology*, Butterworth-Heinemann, Boston, 1995, with permission.

People with emptying problems (inability to urinate at all or incomplete bladder emptying) usually have a bladder that simply doesn't work because it doesn't get the right messages from the brain or spinal cörd. The best treatment is intermittent catheterization either through the urethra or a continent abdominal stoma. If you have both a storage and emptying problem, treatment needs to be individually tailored to the specifics of your condition.

MULTIPLE SCLEROSIS

Multiple sclerosis (MS) is the most common neurologic disease affecting young and middle-aged adults. It is estimated that there are about 500,000 people in the United States with MS and about 10 new cases are diagnosed per 100,000 people each year. It is most common in the third to fifth decades of life and affects women more commonly than men at a ratio of about 3:1. MS is caused by a degenerative process called demyelination, and therefore, MS is called a demyelating disease. Myelin is a protein that encases nerves like the clear wrapping on packaged foods. This myelin sheath is necessary for transmission of nerve impulses, and demyelination results in impaired nerve conduction, which causes many different kinds of neurologic symptoms. The natural course of MS is variable, but the great majority of patients have mild neurologic abnormalities that tend to get worse and then better over time. In many patients, the symptoms are so mild that they never even know that they have MS. The most severe cases, though, are characterized by chronic progression that may ultimately lead to paralysis.

The most common symptoms of MS are blurred or double vision, numbness and tingling in different parts of the body, muscular weakness, and poor balance. Lower urinary tract symptoms (LUTS) are also very common. They are part of the initial symptoms in about 2% of cases, but are present in about 80% of patients at some time in the course of their disease.

The most common bladder symptoms are urinary frequency, urgency, and urge incontinence that is usually caused by involuntary bladder contractions (detrusor hyperreflexia). Of the patients with detrusor hyperreflexia, more than half also have detrusor–external sphincter dyssynergia (DESD). Remember, DESD is an uncoordinated kind of urination in which during bladder contraction, the sphincter contracts as well. The involuntary bladder contraction causes incontinence, but the sphincter contraction causes a partial blockage to the flow of urine. In women, DESD is mostly a nuisance causing urinary incontinence, but in men it is a serious condition that, if not properly treated, can lead to significant kidney problems.

Since the course of MS is so variable, treatment of bladder symptoms requires careful consideration and a highly individualized approach in each patient. The most effective treatment is predicated on a clear understanding of the underlying causes and this, in turn, requires a detailed evaluation, including urodynamic studies. In general, for patients with MS, therapy should commence with the least invasive kind of treatment such as medications and behavior modification. Surgery, particularly irreversible surgery, should be reserved for patients with stable or progressive disease who have no reasonable hope for recovery and in whom conservative therapy has failed. Most patients with exacerbating and remitting forms of MS will continue in that pattern for long periods of time; these patients are best managed conservatively for as long as possible.

STROKE (CVA, OR CEREBROVASCULAR ACCIDENT)

Stroke has a prevalence of 83 to 160 per 100,000 population, the third most common cause of disability in the USA. The most common causes of stroke are (1) arteriosclerosis resulting in blockage of an artery to the brain, (2) hemorrhage (bleeding into the brain, usually from a ruptured aneurysm), and (3) congenital abnormalities of the blood vessels. The first two conditions are associated with hypertension, diabetes, and high blood cholesterol. Screening for these conditions is an essential component of your annual medical checkup, since stroke is largely preventable if these conditions are held in check.

Immediately after stroke, over half of stroke victims develop urinary frequency, urgency, and urge incontinence due to involuntary bladder contractions, and about one quarter develop an areflexic bladder (one that doesn't contract) and cannot urinate at all. Fortunately, in all but about 10% of these people, there is eventually complete recovery, but sometimes this can take as long as a year. While waiting for recovery, treatment can be very difficult, particularly if the stroke has interfered with communication skills. This is often a very frustrating and depressing time for the person.

Unless there are concomitant conditions such as a blockage by the prostate (in men) or stress incontinence (in women), the only clinical problem is that of urinary frequency, urgency, and/or urge incontinence. Some people are aware of the involuntary bladder contraction, which they perceive as an urge to void. Once aware of it, some of these people can actu-

ally abort the involuntary bladder contraction by contracting their sphincter. These people usually complain of urinary frequency and urgency.
Others are aware of the involuntary bladder contraction, but cannot abort
it; they complain of urinary frequency, urgency, and urge incontinence.
Still others are totally unaware and merely find themselves wet. The degree of concern that the patient exhibits about his urinary symptoms is an
important variable, which is usually a function of the neurologic deficit. If
patients are unconcerned about incontinence, it is very unlikely that any
form of medical or surgical therapy will be effective, but if patients are
aware and concerned, the majority of these patients can be cured or
helped. The reason for this is that most of the therapies for involuntary
bladder contractions involve considerable interaction between patient and
doctor. If you have involuntary bladder contractions, one of the most effective therapies is behavior modification. This requires you to keep a
voiding diary, to regulate your fluid intake, and to urinate at predeter-
mined times, based on a review of your diary. Obviously, if you are unaware, unconcerned, or unmotivated, you will not be able to adhere to
such a schedule.

In addition to the effects of the stroke itself, other preexisting urologic
conditions may compound the clinical problem. Men over the age of 40
years have a 5–10% incidence of benign prostatic obstruction; by age 80
the incidence rises to approximately 80%. Women have an increasing incidence of stress incontinence with advancing age. It is particularly important to keep these factors in mind because in many patients the neurologic
abnormality may precipitate the development of symptoms due to the underlying urologic abnormality.

Initial therapy should be conservative, minimally invasive, and completely reversible whenever possible. At first, during the few days after
the stroke, patients are usually managed with an indwelling catheter.
Once this critical stage has passed, it is prudent to switch to intermittent
catheterization. Most patients will be able to void on their own at this time
and in many patients the intermittent catheterization can be discontinued
within a day or two. Many other patients will urinate OK, but develop incontinence due to involuntary bladder contractions. Of course, urinary
tract infection should be excluded or treated and then a decision needs to
be made about further therapy. Some patients will be best managed with
prompted voiding, a form of behavior modification. Prompted voiding is
really little more than reminding the person when to urinate. It is best
done if a voiding diary is kept. The diary is kept for 24 hours by a caregiver and the time and amount of each urination and incontinent episode
are recorded. With simple logic it is possible to plan the best times for the

patient to urinate in order to stay dry. For example, if the diary shows that the person is perfectly dry for one and a half hours at a time, but is incontinent whenever he or she waits longer than that, simply reminding or "prompting" him or her to urinate every one and a half hours may be all that is needed for continence. Alternatively, by looking at the diary, it may be possible to change the person's drinking habits so that the amount of urine in the bladder is more predictable, allowing the person to void according to a schedule. The caregiver then reminds or assists the patient to void at the designated time. Many patients regain full bladder control over the course of weeks or months when this technique is used.

For people with persistent symptoms, it is best to initiate rational treatment based on a clear understanding of the underlying cause of the symptoms. For most people, this requires urodynamic testing. When the basic problem is involuntary bladder contractions due to the neurologic condition, most physicians begin treatment using anticholinergics such as oxybutynin (Ditropan) or tricyclic antidepressant medications such as imipramine (Tofranil), provided that the patient empties his or her bladder. However, I believe that behavior modification should be tried first because not only is it more physiological, but it has a greater success rate and, when effective, it actually cures the problem instead of masking symptoms. If neither of these therapies is effective, the most reasonable short-term solution is the liberal use of absorbent pads or, failing that, an indwelling bladder catheter until the neurologic condition shows no further signs of recovery. If there has been no recovery one year after the initial injury, in carefully selected patients augmentation cystoplasty or urinary diversion may be considered.

PARKINSON'S DISEASE

Parkinson's disease (PD) is a degenerative neurologic disorder that is usually characterized by a slowly progressive course. The classic symptoms consist of slow movements (called bradykinesia), a resting tremor, and stiffness of muscles, called skeletal rigidity. The tremor is a rapid shaking back and forth of the hands at rest, but oddly, the tremor completely stops once the person reaches for something or voluntarily moves the hands. The PD patient has a classic appearance: a slightly stooped posture, an expressionless face, tremors of the hands, and a shuffling gait. In more severe cases, it is very difficult for them to start any movement and once moving, it's hard to stop. The annual prevalence of PD is estimated at 100–150 cases per 100,000 population.

PD is caused by degeneration of a part of the brain called the sub-stantia nigra. This results in a deficiency of a chemical neurotransmitter called dopamine and a predominance of another neurotransmitter called acetylcholine. It is the imbalance between these two chemicals that is thought to cause the symptoms in PD. Approximately 25% of patients with PD have lower urinary tract symptoms (LUTS). The most common symptom is urge incontinence due to involuntary bladder contractions (detrusor hyperreflexia). However, people with PD who have persistent LUTS pose a considerable diagnostic and therapeutic challenge because many of them have other conditions that can exactly mimic the symp-toms due to PD. For example, most older men have an enlarged prostate (benign prostatic hyperplasia, or BPH) and BPH causes identical LUTS symptoms to PD. Further, many people with PD have also had strokes and the LUTS in people with strokes is similar to those due to PD. For all these reasons, it is most difficult to determine whether the symptoms are due to PD, stroke, or BPH. Further, even when a blockage due to the prostate is proven in men with PD, prostate surgery is effective in only about half. In the remainder, persistent symptoms of involuntary blad-der contractions are a cause of significant morbidity and after surgery these patients are even more difficult to treat. Unfortunately, I do not have a simple solution for this complicated clinical problem, but ad-monish you not to undergo surgery without careful consideration of all the options. The fact that half of PD patients do derive benefit from surgery compounds the problem even further because there are no clear guidelines to predict who will benefit and who will get worse. And re-member, the other half derive no benefit from surgery and some even get worse.

INJURIES TO THE NERVOUS SYSTEM

Brain Injuries

Injuries to the brain are most often the result of automobile accidents. Approximately 50,000–75,000 new cases of brain injury are seen in the USA each year (a prevalence of 10–15 per 100,000 population). Not all brain injuries affect the lower urinary tract, but when they do, the vast majority result in involuntary bladder contractions. Traumatic injuries af-fect young people and middle-aged adults much more often than the el-derly. Hence, there is a much lower likelihood of concomitant urologic conditions such as BPH in men or stress incontinence in women. As in stroke, the degree of concern that patients exhibit about their urinary

symptoms is an important variable, and is usually a function of the neurologic deficit (the degree of brain injury). In the person who is unconcerned or unaware, treatment is not very successful, because so much of
the treatment requires a cooperative, motivated patient.

In many instances, the brain injury improves dramatically within the
first few months after injury; in fact, there may be complete recovery a
year or more afterward. Accordingly, initial therapy should be conservative, minimally invasive, and completely reversible whenever possible.
Treatment guidelines are identical to those for stroke and should be based
on a clear understanding of the underlying cause of the symptoms as discussed above.

Spinal Cord Injury

Spinal cord injury afflicts approximately 250,000 Americans (300 per
100,000 population). There are about 3 per 100,000 new injuries each year.
The most common cause of spinal cord injury is automobile accidents
(40%), followed by other kinds of accidents, such as diving accidents
(30%). Gunshot wounds account for another 20% and the remainder are
caused by miscellaneous conditions such as spinal cord tumors, transverse myelitis (an inflammation or infection of the spinal cord that is usually due to a virus), and complications from surgery. The vast majority of
spinal cord injuries result from a broken neck with subsequent damage to
the spinal cord. The spinal cord, which contains the nerve fibers that connect the brain to all other parts of the body, runs through the center of the
spine (backbone) through a tunnel-like structure called the spinal canal.
The spinal canal is surrounded by the bones of the spine, which are very
strong and offer stable protection to the spinal cord, so only with severe
trauma are the spinal cord and its nerves injured.

After spinal cord trauma, there are three fairly distinct phases—
spinal shock, the recovery stage, and the stable phase—accompanied by a
progression of urologic conditions.

Spinal Shock

Immediately after spinal cord injury, there is usually a period of
spinal shock during which there is a complete (flaccid) paralysis, which
means that the muscles below the injury are completely paralyzed and
flabby. Reflexes to the paralyzed muscles are also absent. An example of a
reflex is the knee jerk reflex, which your doctor checks by tapping with a
rubber reflex hammer on the tendon just below the knee cap. If the knee

jerk reflex is present, the lower leg moves forward involuntarily. In the period during spinal shock, all such reflexes are lost. Another kind of paralysis, called spastic paralysis—which is usually caused by a brain injury or stroke—also develops during the spinal shock phase of spinal cord injury. In this kind of paralysis, the reflexes are intact and the muscles are stiff or spastic, as opposed to flabby. Even though they are spastic, these muscles are also paralyzed, which means there is no voluntary movement.

During spinal shock the bladder, like the other muscles below the injury, is completely paralyzed. It does not contract and the patient is unable to urinate at all. There are few treatment options at this time—the bladder must be emptied with a catheter. Since spinal cord injury is often associated with other serious injuries, during the acute critical stage, it is important to monitor the urinary output hour by hour. For this reason, an indwelling catheter is usually used—one that is left in the bladder continuously. In most instances, the catheter is passed through the urethra and held in place with a little fluid-filled balloon at the end of the catheter. Sometimes, if there has been emergency abdominal or bladder surgery because of other injuries sustained at the same time as the spinal cord injury, a suprapubic catheter is left in place. A suprapubic catheter is placed directly into the bladder and comes through a small opening in the lower abdomen.

The duration of spinal shock is variable. In most instances reflex bladder activity (bladder contraction) reappears after six to twelve weeks, but in some cases it may take as long as six to twelve months or more. I have even seen the bladder recover five years after injury! Once the patient is medically stable, the indwelling catheter should be removed and intermittent catheterization instituted at four- to six-hour intervals until the bladder begins to show signs of recovery. Bladder recovery usually becomes evident by the development of urinary incontinence or the return of bladder sensations and voluntary urination.

Recovery Stage

Once the patient has recovered from spinal shock, it is important that he or she undergoes urodynamic tests so that the doctor can make an accurate diagnosis as to the cause of the bladder symptoms. During the recovery period, it is usually best to continue intermittent catheterization, with or without medications and absorbent pads, until the patient has reached the stable phase. This can be a very frustrating period for the patient because it may be difficult to maintain continence since the bladder is in a state of flux while it is healing.

Stable Phase

Most people with a broken neck develop involuntary bladder contractions (detrusor hyperreflexia) and most have detrusor–external
sphincter dyssynergia (DESD, discussed above). Treatment of detrusor–
external sphincter dyssynergia depends on the sex of the patient and the
level of the neurologic lesion. Paraplegia refers to paralysis of the lower
half of the body and results from spinal cord injury below the neck, usually in the middle of the spinal cord, which is called the thoracic or lumbar spinal region. Quadriplegia refers to paralysis of all four extremities
and usually results from injuries to the neck (in the cervical spine). In
paraplegics, the usual goal of therapy is to paralyze the bladder (to keep
it from contracting involuntarily and causing incontinence) and manage
the patient with intermittent catheterization. If anticholinergic medications and the tricyclic antidepressants are ineffective at paralyzing the
bladder, augmentation cystoplasty is almost always successful (see Chapter 20). Many paraplegic and quadriplegic women and some quadriplegic
men are unable to catheterize themselves in a wheelchair. In these people,
it is sometimes advisable to perform an operation to obliterate the urethra
(so urine can't leak out), enlarge (augment) the bladder using the intestine
(to allow it to store urine at low pressure), and create a continent abdominal stoma that the patient can catheterize (to empty the bladder and stay
dry). If the person is unable to catheterize himself or herself at all, urinary
diversion or an augmentation cystoplasty with an incontinent abdominal
stoma may be considered.

All of these therapies can be expected to result in a patient who is
confidently dry and does not have to use absorbent pads or indwelling
catheters. In men with DESD, there is another alternative—surgery that
abolishes or bypasses the obstruction caused by the sphincter contractions. These surgeries—external sphincterotomy and urethral stents—are
discussed in the next section on quadriplegic men.

Sometimes, after spinal cord injury, the bladder never recovers and
does not contract at all. If that happens it is said to be areflexic. If it never
contracts, normal urination is not possible and the patient is said to be in
urinary retention. This occurs most often with low spinal cord injuries (to
the lumbar and sacral part of the spinal cord) that involve the sacral micturition center (SMC). Occasionally patients with cervical or thoracic lesions (upper spinal cord injury) develop persistent detrusor areflexia.
Some of these patients have actually sustained two or more spinal cord injuries, one of which involves the SMC. Detrusor areflexia is best managed
by intermittent catheterization.

Quadriplegic Men

Most quadriplegic men have DESD and most are unable to catheterize themselves through the urethra. For these people there are several options. The most common treatment is an operation called external sphincterotomy and condom catheter drainage. In this procedure, the sphincter muscle (which is causing the blockage) is cut using a cystoscopic surgical instrument or a laser. This relieves the blockage, but the patient becomes even more incontinent. The incontinence is managed with a condom catheter, a silastic (soft, pliable plastic) or rubber condom that goes around the penis and is held in place with adhesive or Velcro. The tip of the condom is attached to tubing that goes to a drainage bag, usually worn on the leg, which needs to be emptied periodically throughout the day. External sphincterotomy should not be performed until it is clear that there is no reasonable chance of further neurologic recovery and that it will be practical for the man to use a condom catheter.

A new approach to DESD is the use of a urethral stent. This is a metal device that looks like a Chinese finger trap. It is placed in the urethra with a cystoscope, bypassing the obstruction caused by the sphincter. The subsequent incontinence must be managed with a condom catheter.

Occasionally, quadriplegic men are able to perform self intermittent catheterization and, if this is the case, they can be treated with medications to paralyze the bladder and allow self intermittent catheterization. If the patient is unable to catheterize himself through the urethra, an augmentation cystoplasty with a continent or incontinent abdominal stoma offers a suitable and safer alternative to urinary diversion.

Quadriplegic Women

Quadriplegic women pose the most difficult clinical challenge. Since there is, as yet, no suitable external drainage device, the only alternative is an indwelling catheter or an operation to create an abdominal stoma for self-catheterization or for use with a urinary drainage bag.

Paraplegics

Treatment of paraplegic patients depends on two factors: (1) what kind of bladder they have and (2) whether they can catheterize themselves. Patients with a damaged sacral micturition center (SMC) (the lower portion of the spinal cord that controls urination) usually develop a large-capacity areflexic bladder that exhibits low pressure. If the patient can do intermittent catheterization, that is by far the best treatment. After a period of time, usually two or more years, some of these patients develop low bladder compliance, a measure of bladder wall stiffness. The stiffer the bladder, the higher the pressure reached as the bladder fills with urine. In practice, when the bladder pressure exceeds 30–40 cm H_2O, the risk for developing urologic complications is exceedingly high. Fortunately, in most patients this risk can be managed simply by increasing the frequency of catheterizations. In some patients anticholinergic medication becomes necessary and, failing this, augmentation cystoplasty is almost always effective provided that the patient remains on intermittent self-catheterization.

Some paraplegic patients have sustained an injury to both the SMC and the sympathetic nerves that innervate the sphincter. Paradoxically, these patients have both incontinence (because the sphincter doesn't work) and urinary retention (because the bladder doesn't work). This is most often seen in injuries of the midportion of the spinal cord, known as the thoracolumbar spine. In men, intermittent catheterization will often control the incontinence, but in women, it may be necessary to perform surgery to repair the sphincter (periurethral collagen injections or a pubovaginal sling as described in Chapter 8). Rarely, collagen injections or an artificial sphincter may be necessary in men.

CONCLUSION

The bladder and sphincter are normally under the control of the nervous system. There are three parts of the nervous system that are primarily responsible—an area in the brain itself (the pontine micturition center) and two in the spinal cord. When there is disruption to the nervous innervation of the lower urinary tract, from disease or injury, control of urination is lost. This can result in uncontrollable urination (incontinence) or in the inability to urinate at all (urinary retention). It can also result in two conditions that pose a serious threat to your health—detrusor–external sphincter dyssynergia (DESD) and low bladder compliance. DESD is an uncoordinated urination caused by involuntary bladder contractions and involuntary sphincter contractions. Involuntary bladder contractions cause incontinence; involuntary sphincter contractions cause a blockage to the flow of urine, which causes high pressure in the bladder. Low bladder compliance is really a stiffness of the bladder wall that also results in high bladder pressure. The high bladder pressure from either of these conditions causes back pressure to the kidneys and, left untreated, leads to kidney damage, stones, infection, and ultimately kidney failure. All of these complications are preventable with early diagnosis and treatment.

The common conditions that cause neurogenic bladder include spinal cord injury, multiple sclerosis, spina bifida, stroke, diabetes mellitus and Parkinson's disease. The symptoms that result from these conditions are treatable, but often intermittent self-catheterization is required. With proper treatment, incontinence can be completely controlled and serious kidney complications prevented. Without proper treatment, though, complications from kidney disease are very common.

18

Aging and the Bladder

... You and I are old;
old age hath yet his honor and his toil;
... Come my friends,
'Tis not too late to seek a newer world,
... and tho'
we are not now that strength which in old days moved
heaven and earth, that which we are, we are,
One equal temper of heroic heart,
made weak by time and fate, but strong in will,
to strive to seek to find and not to yield.

—ALFRED, LORD TENNYSON, *Ulysses*

Things break. Old things break more often than new things. The hardest thing to break, though, is the human spirit. As long as you've got your mind and your will, there are successful treatments for nearly every bladder problem that afflicts the elderly.

—ANONYMOUS

INTRODUCTION

As you get older, things don't work as well as they used to, and the urinary tract is no exception. Although there have been many studies on the effects of aging on the lower urinary tract, the results have not yielded any straightforward conclusions. It is not clear, for example, whether it is the aging process itself or the accompanying diseases and afflictions of older age (e.g., prostatic growth in men and loss of estrogen in women) that account for the symptoms. Regardless of the cause, a number of generalities apply to both men and women as they age. First, with advancing age, there

239

is a tendency toward increased frequency of urination, nocturia (getting up at night to urinate), and a decrease in the force and strength of the urinary stream. Second, in men, the prostate begins to hypertrophy (the size and number of prostate cells increase), resulting in prostatic enlargement known as benign prostatic hyperplasia (BPH). In most men BPH is associated with a blockage in the urethra and may cause a number of lower urinary tract symptoms (LUTS). Third, in women, after menopause, the level of the female hormone estrogen declines precipitously. This results in many symptoms, including hot flashes and vaginal dryness. Finally, in women, the sphincter muscle often weakens, resulting in incontinence.

For the majority of people, though, aging is associated with bladder symptoms that are barely noticeable and cause no concerns at all. However, when caused by disease processes such as prostate problems in men and gynecologic problems in women, the symptoms may be more troublesome and require treatment. In elderly patients, the approach to treatment is nearly identical to that in younger people; you can look back in the relevant chapters for a more detailed explanation. With aging though, other problems might arise that generally do not in themselves cause symptoms, but can exacerbate already existing ones and make them much more difficult to deal with.

Neil Resnick, Associate Professor of Medicine at Harvard Medical School and Chief of Gerontology at the Brigham and Women's Hospital in Boston, is the foremost authority in the United States on aging and the bladder. He is an exemplary and caring physician and a passionate advocate for a thoughtful, humanistic approach to health care in the elderly. He emphasizes the importance of realizing that the maladies that accompany old age are not caused by aging per se; rather, they are simply afflictions or illnesses that occur in old age. That means that we should approach each older person as if he or she has an underlying disease or condition that needs treatment, not as an old person with symptoms due to age. For example, prostate cancer is not caused by the aging process, but, for practical purposes, the older you are, the more likely you are to be afflicted by it. Testicular cancer, on the other hand, is seen almost exclusively in boys and young men, yet no one would ever say that testicular cancer is caused by youth. Fortunately, for the majority of conditions, there are effective treatments to prevent bladder symptoms from impacting people's lifestyles.

Dr. Resnick points out that when an older person complains of lower urinary tract symptoms, it is important to go through a checklist of possible contributing factors that can, if treated, often relieve the bladder symptoms. These include many of the afflictions that are more common in old age such as the following.

1. Physical limitations of mobility due to such things as arthritis, Parkinson's disease, or stroke
2. Neurologic conditions such as Parkinson's disease, stroke, and senility
3. Constipation
4. Endocrine diseases such as diabetes and hypothyroidism
5. The effects of menopause in women
6. Benign prostatic hyperplasia in men
7. Depression
8. Side effects of medications

The diagnostic evaluation of lower urinary tract symptoms begins with your doctor doing a history and physical examination, emphasizing the subtle first beginnings of the conditions alluded to above. You should be prepared to give a detailed account of your present and past symptoms, your past medical history, previous surgeries, other illnesses or conditions, and a listing of all current medications and dosages. Your doctor should do a physical examination, and a urine sample should be obtained for analysis and culture.

If the urinalysis and culture indicate a urinary tract infection it should be treated. Even in older people, urinary tract infection is still the most common cause of bladder symptoms. If hematuria (blood in the urine) is found, you'll need an evaluation for that including cystoscopy and a kidney X ray as discussed in Chapter 4. Once urinary tract infection has been excluded or treated and hematuria evaluated (present), a voiding diary should be obtained recording the time and amount of each urination and the associated symptoms. Urinary flow rate (uroflow) and postvoid residual (the amount of urine remaining in your bladder after you've finished voiding) should be obtained as well. Based on this evaluation, the need for further testing can be assessed.

INFECTION

Bladder and prostate infections are the most common cause of bladder symptoms in the elderly and, in old age, men and women are affected about equally. In most cases, the diagnosis is obvious because the person experiences the usual symptoms of urinary tract infection (UTI)—urinary frequency, urgency, burning, and pain. Not infrequently, though, the symptoms are more subtle. The person may complain only of urinary frequency or getting up at night to urinate or even incontinence. There may be no pain or burning at all. Sometimes, there may even be blood in the urine (hematuria). That is why it is so important to do a urinalysis and culture as part of the initial evaluation of all people with LUTS. Although UTI is the most common cause of bladder symptoms in older people, the infection itself is often caused by another condition. Even after appropriate antibiotic treatment and eradication of the bacteria, there may be persistent symptoms. For example, a man with prostatic obstruction may develop a UTI because of incomplete bladder emptying and after treatment of the infection he may have persistent symptoms due to the underlying blockage.

It is particularly important to realize that UTIs are often accompanied by hematuria. Conversely, hematuria may actually be mistaken for a UTI. After the infection has been treated, it is important that the urinalysis be repeated and if the hematuria persists, a careful evaluation to exclude more serious causes such as bladder and prostate cancer is a necessary part of the evaluation. Further, if it turns out that the infections seem to recur, even after adequate treatment, a careful search should be made to see if there is an underlying cause for the infection. In men, this is most likely to be due to an enlarged prostate; in women, it is often the effects of decreased estrogen output after the menopause.

PROSTATE PROBLEMS IN MEN

As alluded to above, BPH is nearly a universal accompaniment of the aging process in men. BPH is accompanied by lower urinary tract symptoms (LUTS) in the majority of men, but in most the symptoms are mild and do not require any treatment at all. If LUTS are bothersome enough, though, you may want to consider treatment and, furthermore, there are certain conditions in which treatment is necessary. Treatment *is necessary* if (1) you are unable to urinate at all (urinary retention), (2) there are recurring UTIs, or (3) there is kidney failure due to the blockage. There are usually no symptoms of kidney failure at all (until the very end stages). The only way of determining if there is a significant enough blockage to cause kidney failure is to do an imaging study of the kidney. Imaging studies of the kidney include renal ultrasound, abdominal CAT scan (computerized axial tomography), or abdominal MRI (magnetic resonance imaging).

Fortunately, no matter how bad the symptoms are, there is almost always an effective therapy. The most effective treatments include medications—alpha-adrenergic blocking agents such as terazocin (Hytrin), doxazocin (Cardura), and prazosin (Minipres)—and prostate surgery. Many new and less invasive treatments are still in the clinical investigation stage, as discussed in more detail in Chapter 13.

GYNECOLOGIC PROBLEMS IN WOMEN

As men get older, the prostate enlarges (benign prostatic hyperplasia); as women get older, the uterus shrinks (uterine atrophy). In the grand scheme of things, that might make sense, but the logic of it eludes me. The uterus shrinks because estrogen production by the ovaries ceases after menopause. Lack of estrogen causes an increased tendency toward osteoporosis and heart disease; it causes dryness of the eyes and atrophy of the vagina, uterus, cervix, and tissues around the urethra, which may cause vaginal dryness, itching, and painful sex. Further, the muscles and ligaments that hold the bladder, uterus, and rectum in place may begin to weaken causing incontinence and *prolapse*, which means to slide forward or downward. Genital prolapse refers to a prolapse of the bladder, uterus, or rectum through the vagina. The medical term for prolapsed bladder is *cystocele*, and for prolapsed rectum, *rectocele*.

Although there is tremendous controversy about the use of estrogen in older women, the overall effects are quite beneficial. In women with infection or incontinence, administration of estrogen, either in the pill form or as a vaginal suppository, often is effective in reducing the chances of further infection. In addition, it may also help with incontinence. The main risk is that women treated with estrogen alone have a higher chance of developing cancer of the uterus. However, if it's combined with progesterone there is no additional risk of developing uterine cancer and it's actually quite safe. Of course, if you've already had a hysterectomy, then there is no chance of developing uterine cancer. The second risk from estrogen is a possible increase in the chances of developing breast cancer, but that risk appears to be limited to women that already have a predisposition because of genes or a family history of breast cancer. Overall, in my judgment, the medical benefits of estrogen (decreased heart disease, decreased osteoporosis, decreased atrophy) far outweigh the potential harm in most women. From a clinical standpoint, the major downside of hormone replacement therapy (estrogen alone or estrogen and progesterone) are the side effects, particularly those associated with added progesterone. The decision whether or not to utilize hormone replacement therapy is a highly individualized one and you should discuss this in detail with your doctor.

For women with prolapse, there are a number of effective treatments. If the prolapse is mild, pelvic floor exercises (Kegel exercises; see Chapter 8) may be effective. For more severe cases a pessary may be used. A pessary, as noted before, is an appliance, like a diaphragm, that is placed in the vagina to hold the prolapsed organ in place. Pessaries come in many shapes and sizes, the most common shape being like a donut. If you want to consider a pessary, it is necessary to have your doctor evaluate you and fit it to you. Most women can insert and remove the pessary by themselves, but some cannot. If you are unable to remove the pessary, it is safe to leave it in place and have your doctor clean it, inspect the vagina, and replace it every three months. If a pessary is not appealing to you, you may want to consider surgery. Except in rare instances, when the prolapse is so bad that it causes a blockage to the ureters, severe bleeding, pain, or the inability to urinate at all, surgery is entirely elective.

MEDICATION

A number of medications can cause bladder problems. If you are having bladder problems one of the first things you should do is discuss with your doctor whether any of the medications you are taking might be causing you symptoms. For example, over-the-counter cold remedies and decongestants often contain substances that tighten the sphincter (alpha-adrenergic agonists), like phenylpropanolamine. In men with BPH or women with a weak bladder, this can make it difficult to urinate and even cause urinary retention (the inability to urinate at all). Medications with anticholinergic effects also make it more difficult to urinate because they can partially or completely paralyze the bladder. Agents with anticholinergic properties include antihistamines, antidepressants, antipsychotics, opiates, gastrointestinal tract antispasmodics, and medications to counter Parkinson's disease. Sedative hypnotics and alcohol depress general behavior and the sensorium (the intellectual functions); they may depress bladder contractility and reduce attention to bladder cues. Calcium channel blockers for hypertension or coronary artery disease are smooth muscle relaxants and can facilitate bladder storage, and may cause urinary retention and overflow incontinence. When you first start a diuretic it causes you to urinate more frequently because your kidneys make more urine. However, if your doctor has instructed you to take diuretics on a daily basis, after a few days or a week, you should reach a steady state and begin to urinate in normal amounts again.

DIABETES

Diabetes, particularly when unrecognized or poorly treated, is a major cause of lower urinary tract symptoms. There are a number of different ways that diabetes can cause bladder symptoms. First, when the diabetes is not well treated with diet or medications, the blood sugar level can get very high, driving up the thirst mechanism so that you drink a lot. The more you drink, the more you urinate, so most patients with poorly controlled diabetes have a large urinary output that results in frequency of urination. Another problem that diabetics have, though, is neuropathy. This means that the nerves to the bladder (and other parts of the body) have been damaged by a process caused demyelination. When this happens, conduction along the nerve is delayed or impaired and the organ innervated by the nerve, in this case the bladder and the sphincter, don't work normally. This results in a condition known as diabetic cystopathy. The first sign of diabetic cystopathy is reduced bladder sensations. When this happens you no longer feel the urge to urinate at normal volumes. In turn, the bladder must become more and more distended until you feel the urge to urinate. At first, these patients void less frequently than normal. The volume of each urination is larger as long as the bladder continues to work normally, which it does at the beginning. Over time, though, the bladder wall becomes stretched, the muscle weakens, and it becomes increasingly difficult for you to empty your bladder. Since bladder sensations are also impaired most patients are not even aware of any symptoms at all. Eventually, unless there is treatment, residual urine builds up in the bladder, leading to recurring infections, marked difficulty urinating, and ultimately kidney failure.

Treatment begins with an accurate diagnosis obtained by history, urinalysis (a positive glucose), and blood tests. Once diabetes is recognized it is treated. This is generally done by a general practitioner, an internist, or an endocrinologist. Treatment may be by diet alone, by medications that regulate the blood sugar in a pill form, or finally by different regimens of insulin by injection. Proper control of the diabetes should take care of the bladder problem. However, if diabetic cystopathy has already set in, it is generally not reversible by the medications and will require specific treatment. Since your sensations don't allow you to feel the need to urinate, it may be necessary for you to "void by the clock." This means that you urinate on a schedule based on the times and estimated amount of urine in the bladder. This is best done in conjunction with the behavior therapy program wherein voiding diaries are utilized. If the bladder has been irreparably damaged it may be necessary to do intermittent self-catheterization. Finally, in men, there may be an element of prostatic obstruction combined with the diabetes that also needs treatment (see Chapter 13).

DECREASED MOBILITY

Once the urge to urinate is felt, most people can comfortably wait until they get to the bathroom. However, if you've just broken your hip, or you have Parkinson's disease, or your back is out of whack, it is not so easy. In many older people the warning time (the time from when they first get the urge to urinate to the time that it is quite severe) is decreased. If you have decreased mobility you might not be able to get to the bathroom in time. In most instances, this is a temporary problem that abates once mobility is restored to normal. If, for whatever reason, the condition is not a temporary one, it must be dealt with, and there are many ways to do so. One of the most common problems that people with physical limitations have is the inability to get out of a chair quickly and get to the bathroom. In some instances the problem may be more with the chair than with the person. If you are sitting, and your buttocks are lower than your knees, getting up may require more strength than you have. If that is the case, it is a fairly simple matter to sit on a pillow or to buy a chair that allows you to sit with your knees level with or lower than your buttocks. In that way getting up and getting to the bathroom will be an order-of-magnitude easier.

If mobility is restricted to the point where it is simply impractical to get to the bathroom fast enough, a bedside commode for women or a urinal for men can be used as a temporary or a long-term solution. In rare instances, it may be necessary for a man to use a condom catheter or a woman to have an indwelling catheter until the disabling condition remits.

NEUROLOGIC CONDITIONS

There are a number of neurologic conditions that occur more frequently with advancing age. These include stroke, Parkinson's disease, and Alzheimer's disease. After suffering a stroke (cerebrovascular accident) most people develop incontinence. Fortunately, in the majority, there is complete recovery over a matter of weeks or months; rarely it may take a year. In many instances, the incontinence is actually due to an unrecognized urinary tract infection that is contracted when the patient is catheterized during the acute treatment of the stroke. This emphasizes the need for careful evaluation, beginning with urinalysis and culture, whenever LUTS occur, even if the symptoms seem to be related to something else. If after suffering a stroke, incontinence or other LUTS persist for more than a few months, it is important that a urologist be consulted. In most instances, after an accurate diagnosis is attained, effective treatment is available.

As they get older, some people become senile or develop Alzheimer's disease. Neither of these conditions by itself affects urination. In fact, most people with senility or Alzheimer's disease are not incontinent unless they have some other condition, like BPH in men or stress incontinence in women. In the absence of other conditions, the most common cause of incontinence in these people is that they are simply unconcerned about when and where they urinate. This is obviously a most difficult condition to treat and about the best that we can do is to use a technique called prompted voiding with such people. This means that a dedicated person, a caregiver, family member, etc. helps the person to the bathroom periodically throughout the day. If one pays careful attention and figures out about how often the person urinates it is usually possible to bring him or her to the bathroom before such time as urination would occur in a socially unacceptable place. Although getting the person to the toilet is generally effective, it does take a considerable expenditure of time and effort on the part of the caregiver. It can be very frustrating and it can be very expensive. If toileting is ineffective, about the best you can do is to use plenty of diapers and pads. Medications and other treatments are ineffective because there is nothing wrong with the person except for their unconcern about urination.

Parkinson's disease is another common neurologic disease of old age that commonly affects the bladder. The usual problem is that the bladder contracts involuntarily, causing the person to urinate without control. In men, there is usually an accompanying BPH problem that might also need attention (this topic is covered in much more detail in Chapter 17).

CONCLUSION

Lower urinary tract symptoms (LUTS) in older people are not caused by aging per se, but by the many afflictions that are more common in old age. Further, if LUTS should occur, it is often possible to find an underlying remediable cause and an effective treatment that restores normal or near-normal functioning. In older people with physical or cognitive abnormalities, it may be necessary to enlist the services of a caregiver to assist with these bladder problems, but often simple environmental changes may be all that is needed, such as putting a chair close to the bathroom with a high enough seat so that the patient can easily get out of the chair without assistance.

19

Fistula
A Hole in the Bladder

INTRODUCTION

A *fistula* is an abnormal passage or connection between a hollow body cavity, like the bladder, and the surface of the body. A *vesicovaginal fistula* connects the bladder with the vagina; a *urethrovaginal fistula* connects the urethra to the vagina. Vesicovaginal and urethrovaginal fistulas result in severe urinary incontinence because there is uncontrollable leakage of urine through the fistula, which bypasses the urethra and the sphincter. Imagine that the bladder is like an inflated balloon and the sphincter is like the knot that keeps the air from leaking out; a fistula is like a hole in the balloon. Fistulas are almost always the result of complications from pelvic surgery (hysterectomy, prolapse repair, or anti-incontinence surgery) or from childbirth injuries. Rarely, they may be caused by pelvic cancer.

In the industrial countries of the world, obstetric injuries are exceedingly uncommon, but in the third world, particularly in Africa and Asia, childbirth injuries continue to exact a toll of enormous social and medical consequence. In the third world, fistulas are most often the result of prolonged labor, 24 hours or more, particularly when the fetus is very large compared to the size of the mother's pelvis (maternal–fetal disproportion). When there is such a disproportion, the head of the baby becomes stuck in the vaginal canal and presses on the bladder and urethra. If this lasts too long a time, the blood vessels in the mother's vagina are compressed and the tissues cannot get enough oxygen. Without oxygen, the individual cells of the tissues begin to die, called ischemic necrosis. Ischemic necrosis destroys the tissues between the bladder and vagina, resulting in a vesicovaginal or urethrovaginal fistula, which cannot heal because of the damaged blood supply.

In the countries of the third world there are special hospitals, called fistula hospitals, where a few dedicated surgeons devote their time to the surgical repair of these terrible maladies. The compassion and surgical skills of these doctors are extraordinary; to me they represent the pinnacle of devotion and personal sacrifice that exemplify being a doctor. The society of mankind owes them all a debt of gratitude, and as a surgeon myself, I add my personal thanks to Anna Ward, a missionary surgeon in Nigeria, to John Kelly in Zambia, to John Lawson, who trained them both and has retired to his home in the United Kingdom, to T. S. Ghosh and J. O. Martey in Ghana, and to Katherine and Reginald Hamlin in Ethiopia and Abo Abo in the Sudan. Thomas Elkins, an American gynecologist, has traveled to Africa nearly ever year since 1975, at first to learn and then to teach fistula surgery. Tom is a good friend and now Professor and Head of Gynecology at Johns Hopkins. He is surely one of the most experienced fistula surgeons in America.

The high success rate of these surgeons in treating the most extensive of childbirth fistulas is well known. However, when the sphincter and urethra are involved (urethrovaginal fistulas), a high incidence of persistent incontinence may ensue that, if not cured, becomes a devastating problem that almost invariably results in social ostracism and a lonely life of isolation for these mothers who are little more than children themselves.

Surgical treatment of these terrible injuries has become a special interest of mine. I have learned that by repairing the incontinence at the same time that the fistula is surgically repaired, it is possible to cure both the fistula and the incontinence in over 90% of women, provided that a tissue graft bringing in a new blood supply (a Martius graft) is done in conjunction with a pubovaginal sling. I'll discuss what these words mean after describing how the surgeries are done.

In the industrialized countries of the world, like the USA, Canada, and western Europe, fistulas usually are the result of surgical complications from relatively simple operations such as anti-incontinence procedures, hysterectomy, prolapse surgery, or urethral diverticulectomy. In addition, if not properly cared for, the injudicious use of indwelling urethral catheters may result in pressure necrosis, in other words, tissue death, of the urethra. This is most commonly seen in quadriplegic or paraplegic women, but is occasionally encountered in otherwise normal women who have had a prolonged recovery after a devastating illness or injury. This form of injury is particularly disconcerting since it is entirely preventable by routine hygiene and observation. Rarely, urethrovaginal or vesicovaginal fistula may result from a laceration of the urethra and/or vesical neck sustained after trauma to the pelvis, particularly when there has been a fracture of the pubic bone. Rarely there may be local invasion of these tissues from cancer of the pelvis or damage from radiation treatment that results in a fistula.

Regardless of the cause of the fistula, the consequences to the patient are devastating and the diagnostic and therapeutic challenges to the surgeon are considerable. Effective treatment begins with an accurate diagnosis, and diagnosis begins with a high index of suspicion on the part of the physician. Sadly, many, if not most, fistulas are initially misdiagnosed because the symptoms are attributed to some other cause. A high index of suspicion means that the doctor should suspect fistula whenever a woman complains of urinary incontinence shortly after childbirth, vaginal surgery of any type, or hysterectomy. Further, the doctor should be suspicious of fistula in any woman who complains of incontinence but in whom, on examination, urine is not seen to leak from the urethra.

As I discussed in Chapter 8, when a woman complains of incontinence, the sine qua non of diagnosis is for the doctor to actually witness the incontinence and see the urine leak from the urethra. If this simple axiom is followed, urinary fistulas should be correctly diagnosed in the vast majority of patients. The most common symptom of a urinary fistula is a constant or nearly constant leakage of urine, both day and night. Some women with small fistulas urinate fairly normally even though there is a continuous leakage; others leak so much that there is never enough in the bladder for them to urinate at all. In many fistula patients, the leakage is so bad that they constantly soak through incontinence pads even though they are changed frequently throughout the day.

In the majority of patients the diagnosis will be obvious if your doctor does a physical examination when you have a full bladder. If you develop incontinence after childbirth or one of the operations listed above, you should be examined by your doctor, preferably with a full bladder. He or she should examine the vagina looking for the sources of the urinary leakage. If the leakage is not seen, the doctor should pass a catheter, fill the bladder, and look again. If the source is still not apparent, he or she might want to put some dye in through the catheter to help visualize the leakage. Rarely, it will be necessary to do an X ray or CAT scan to make the correct diagnosis. Once the diagnosis is confirmed, it is important to make sure that there are not other injuries to the bladder, urethra, or ureters. Once an accurate diagnosis has been made and other injuries excluded, it is time to consider your treatment options.

TREATMENT

For practical purposes, the only treatments for fistulas are surgical. Some doctors recommend that an indwelling catheter be left in place for a prolonged period of time (weeks or months) to give the fistula a chance to heal on its own. Although there have been a few reports of success using this method, most of the time it is unsuccessful and only delays the otherwise inevitable surgery. Further, it is very frustrating for a woman to spend weeks or months with a catheter in place, especially because the catheter usually is ineffective in controlling the leakage and, aside from the liberal use of absorbent pads, there is no good way of keeping her dry.

There are two main types of surgical repair of vesicovaginal fistula— an abdominal repair and a vaginal repair. In general, although there are distinct advantages and disadvantages to each method, the decision to use one or the other is based mostly on the experience and skills of the surgeon. It really doesn't matter whether he or she is a urologist or gynecologist as long as he or she has done plenty of these operations and has a good success rate. In the hands of a skilled surgeon, the chances of success ought to be in the range of 90% or more unless the fistula has been caused by radiation or cancer. Then the success rate is lower, about 60–80%.

How do I actually choose a surgeon? Is it OK to use the doctor who did the operation that caused the problem in the first place?

Finding an experienced surgeon to repair the fistula is not an easy task because fistulas are not very common in industrialized countries and, therefore, there are not many experienced surgeons. I think there are probably experienced surgeons in most large cities and towns, but you really have to check for yourself. If you chose your surgeon carefully in the first place, the chances are that she is highly skilled. If he or she diagnosed your fistula in a timely fashion (within a few days or a week or two) and exhibited care and concern, the best place to start is to discuss the problem with him or her. It may well be that he or she is experienced at performing fistula surgery. If your surgeon is not so experienced, he or she will probably be able to refer you to an experienced surgeon. In general, the more fistula operations a surgeon has performed, the better he or she is, but that's not an infallible rule. You should ask your doctor directly if he or she is experienced, about how many fistula operations he or she has done, and what the success rate has been. There's no way to grade the success of the surgeon and there's no easy way to be sure that you've chosen the right one, but there are commonsense guidelines. Because fistulas are so rare, you're unlikely to find a doctor who has operated on more than a dozen or so. A real expert in industrialized countries may have done a hundred; in Africa a real expert might do thousands of fistula operations. If your doctor has done a dozen and all were successful, that's pretty good; if all failed I'd stay away from that doctor. If her success is over about 80%, that's OK, but I'd rather have a surgeon whose success is well over 90%. If she says that the success rate is 50% or less, I'd look for another. The surgeon really should have a pretty good idea of what her own success rate is because, not only are fistulas rare, but when the surgery is unsuccessful, it's almost always apparent within the first 2–4 weeks.

There are distinct differences between a vaginal and abdominal approach to fistula repair. All things being equal, the vaginal approach is far preferable for a number of reasons. First, the surgery is done completely through the vagina so there is no visible scar. Second, the postoperative recovery is much easier and less painful without an abdominal incision and there is much less chance of wound infection and other complications. Further, blood loss is less and so there is less chance that you will require a blood transfusion.

OK, I'll take the vaginal approach.

It's not quite that simple. In the hands of all but the most expert of fistula surgeons, the abdominal approach probably has a considerably higher success rate. Further, the vaginal approach can result in more vaginal scarring, and it can shorten the vagina and cause painful intercourse (dyspareunia). And in some women, the vagina is simply too small or the fistula is up too high for the surgeon to be able to expose it adequately. In these instances, an abdominal approach should be used. In addition, if there has been an injury to the ureter or the intestine, an abdominal approach is needed so that both surgeries can be accomplished. Further, many urologists are not familiar with the vaginal approach and many gynecologists are not familiar with the abdominal approach. In some instances, at the discretion of your surgeon, it may be better to perform the surgery with a combined approach, through both the vagina and abdomen in order to insure a successful outcome.

No matter which approach is chosen, it is often advisable to bring in a new blood supply to the damaged area to insure that enough oxygen reaches the tissues to allow proper healing. The two most common ways of doing this are with a Martius labial fat pad graft and an omental flap. The Martius flap is used in vaginal repairs. An incision is made over the labia, adjacent to the vaginal opening, and a longitudinal strip of fat, about the width of your index finger, is isolated, with care being taken to preserve the blood vessels feeding the fatty issue. The flap is then tunneled underneath the vaginal wall and placed over the site of the fistula repair. In time, new blood vessels will grow and help nourish the repair.

An omental flap is used in abdominal repairs. The omentum is an apronlike mass of fatty tissue, rich in blood vessels, which hangs down from part of the large intestine called the transverse colon. The ometum has been called "the watchdog of the abdomen" because whenever there is damage or infection to part of the abdomen, the omentum covers it, bringing in a rich blood supply and nourishment to the damaged area and helping it heal.

There is one more approach that I chose to leave till last because I don't really approve of it, and I've never tried it, although I can't say with certainty that it's unwise to try it. It's called fulguration of the fistula tract, a very simple technique that's done with a cystoscope. The fistula is visualized and its edges fulgurated, that is, heated to very high temperatures, which cause the tissue to actually undergo necrosis. The theory is that this will set up an inflammatory reaction around the fistula to which the body will respond by trying to heal it. This doesn't make any sense to me, particularly because it was ischemic necrosis that caused the fistula in the first place. Nevertheless, a few doctors have reported success with this technique.

Timing of Surgery and Preoperative Management

In the past, much controversy surrounded the timing of surgical repair. For decades it had been taught that surgery should be delayed for three to six months or longer to allow adequate time for the tissue to heal and for inflammation and swelling (edema) to subside. Most experts now agree that surgery can be safely performed as soon as the vaginal wound is free of infection and inflammation and the tissues are reasonably pliable (soft). It is almost always possible to perform the surgery within a few weeks after the original surgery.

Management of incontinence while waiting for healing of the vaginal tissue is sometimes a difficult problem. In women with small fistulas, bladder catheter drainage is usually sufficient. If significant leakage occurs with a Foley catheter in place, it is usually best to remove the catheter and manage the incontinence with absorbent pads until the fistula can be surgically repaired.

Postoperative Management

Most fistula surgeons, including me, recommend that a catheter be left in place for a few weeks after surgery until the fistula has had a chance to heal, but a few surgeons only leave a catheter in overnight. It's advisable for the surgeon to check that the fistula has healed before the catheter is removed. This is done by examining the vagina at the site of the fistula repair to be sure that it appears healthy and also by filling the bladder with saline or water or dye and checking that it doesn't leak through the vagina. If healing appears incomplete or if there is still leakage, the catheter should be left in another few weeks, then checked again. For practical purposes, the wound should be well healed by a maximum of four weeks. If there is still leakage at that time, the operation has failed.

Urethrovaginal Fistulas

For women with urethrovaginal fistulas the situation is even more complicated because, in addition to repairing the fistula, it is usually necessary to do an anti-incontinence operation at the same time. One word of caution, though. Not all urethrovaginal fistulas cause a problem and not all have to be surgically repaired. If a urethrovaginal fistula is discovered on examination by your doctor, but you experience no symptoms and have no incontinence, there is no need to repair it at all. However, if there is incontinence, it usually means that the fistula involves not only the urethra, but the sphincter and bladder neck as well.

Surgery to repair these kinds of injuries are much more complicated than the repair of a vesicovaginal fistula and require a very experienced surgeon. First, the surgeon has to repair the urethra, then she has to repair the incontinence. Because she is doing so much surgery in such a small place, it is usually advisable to bring in a new blood supply to insure the best chance for healing. This may be accomplished by a Martius labial fat pad graft, described in the previous section. Despite the complexity of this surgery, in experienced hands, the overall success rate is over 90% with respect to continence and a successful fistula repair.

Historically, there are three different approaches to repairing these injuries: (1) anterior bladder flaps (Tanagaho procedure), (2) posterior bladder flaps (Young–Dees–Leadbetter procedure), and (3) vaginal wall flaps, as I described above. Although these techniques appear to be comparable with respect to repair of the fistula, incontinence persists in about half of the women unless it is repaired at the same time. In my judgment, there is almost never a need to do anything but a vaginal repair combined with pubovaginal sling and Martius flap. I believe that vaginal reconstruction is considerably easier and faster, is much more amenable to concomitant anti-incontinence surgery, and has a much easier recovery with much less complications and less blood loss.

Preoperative Evaluation

Whenever a fistula is diagnosed, one must have a high index of suspicion that there might be other injuries as well that will require surgical repair at the same time as the fistula repair. To overlook these would be a travesty, requiring yet another surgery. There could be a fistula from the ureter to the vagina (a ureterovaginal fistula), an obstruction to the ureter by a suture from the original surgery, or sphincteric incontinence. A careful evaluation to detect these potential conditions should be undertaken prior to surgery so that they may be diagnosed beforehand and repaired at surgery. In order to diagnose these conditions, kidney X rays (IVP and retrograde pyelography) should be performed in all patients whenever possible. Cystoscopy and pelvic examination are also essential.

Further, women with these injuries have usually undergone one or more prior vaginal operations and have urinary incontinence that is very difficult to manage. The vaginal tissues are often very scarred and the blood supply to them may be deficient. Prior to surgery careful examination of the vagina is necessary to determine the actual extent of tissue loss and to assess the availability of local tissue for use in the reconstruction. In most instances there is sufficient tissue in the vagina itself to use for the repair, but if the vaginal tissue is extensively scarred and there is not enough tissue for the repair, other areas such as the labia, the abdomen, and the inner thigh should be evaluated for possible use as tissue grafts.

CONCLUSION

Vesicovaginal and urethrovaginal fistulas (holes in the vagina connected to the bladder and urethra) are rare in industrialized countries, but are common in the third world because of inadequate obstetric care. The only treatment is surgical, and in the hands of experienced surgeons the success rate is very high. Even if the surgery should fail, a second operation or even a third will almost always be successful in expert hands. Whenever a fistula is diagnosed, a careful search for associated injuries to the ureter should be undertaken, and if found, these injuries should be repaired at the same time.

Women with urethrovaginal fistulas have an even more complicated problem because, in addition to the fistula, there is usually an injury to the sphincter as well. In the hands of experts, after a single operation to repair both the fistula and the incontinence, a successful outcome can be achieved in over 90% of women.

20

When All Else Fails
Urinary Reconstruction and Diversion

INTRODUCTION

Despite the best efforts of physicians and surgeons, sometimes the bladder or the urethra has been so severely damaged that it no longer serves its intended purpose and the person is rendered hopelessly incontinent. These circumstances are quite rare and occur almost exclusively in certain specific situations: (1) in people severely disabled by neurologic diseases such as spinal cord injury and multiple sclerosis, (2) when the urethra has been destroyed by surgeries, infection, or tumor, and (3) when the bladder or urethra has been damaged during childbirth. A similar situation occurs when the bladder and/or urethra must be surgically removed as part of a cure for cancer or when there has been extensive damage from radiation treatments for cancer. No matter how severe and hopeless the damage seems, it is still possible for a person to achieve complete continence, remain confidently dry, and lead a normal life after reconstructive surgery. These operations use part of the intestines to replace the functions of the bladder and urethra. There are two kinds of operations that are done: one is called cystoplasty; the other, urinary diversion.

CYSTOPLASTY

Cystoplasty (*cyst* = bladder, *plasty* = to form) is an operation that uses whatever is remaining of the bladder and urethra to reconstruct the basic functions of the bladder and urethra. It's kind of like remodeling a house or adding a room to a house that has become too small for its inhabitants. Cystoplasty is done when the bladder has become either too small to hold enough urine to keep you confidently dry or too stiff (low bladder compliance) to hold urine under low pressure. Some of the conditions that cause the bladder to become too small or to develop low compliance include neurogenic bladder (such as spinal cord injury, spina bifida, and multiple sclerosis), tuberculosis of the bladder, and radiation treatments to the pelvis for cancer.

Cystoplasty is performed by isolating a segment of the intestines, detaching it from the rest of the intestine, and then reconfiguring it into the shape of a half-sphere. The original bladder is opened, and it too is reconfigured into the shape of a half-sphere. The two half-spheres are then sewn together to form the new bladder. The net result of the cystoplasty is a reservoir that stores large volumes of urine at low pressure. Many people are not able to urinate adequately after this procedure and must empty their bladder with intermittent self-catheterization. If the person is not able to catheterize the urethra because of spasticity of the legs (women) or urethral scarring (men), it is possible to construct a continent abdominal stoma (see below) or an ileal chimney.

"ILEAL CHIMNEY"

An ileal chimney is formed by isolating a piece of the small intestine (the ileum). One end is attached to the top of the bladder and the other is brought out to the skin as a stoma. The stoma protrudes about a half inch through the skin and a urostomy drainage bag is used to collect the urine (Figure 1).

All of these operations are major surgeries that usually take two to eight hours or more to perform. Nevertheless, there is not much blood loss associated with them and they are generally quite safe to perform, even in patients with serious neurologic conditions such as spinal cord injury and multiple sclerosis. For most patients the end result is a godsend. People that used to be totally incontinent day and night and who were confined to their homes because of this are able to resume a much more normal day-to-day existence. Once of the most common remarks I hear after this type of surgery is "I wish I had it done ten years ago."

URINARY DIVERSION

Sometimes the bladder and/or urethra are so badly damaged that they cannot be used at all or the bladder must be removed in order to cure

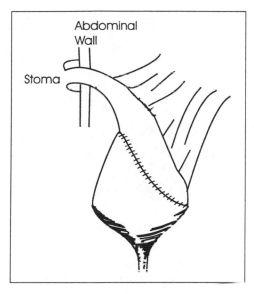

Stoma

Abdominal
Wall

Figure 1. Augmentation cystoplasty with abdominal stoma. The bladder is enlarged with a piece of intestine and an opening (stoma) is made in the skin of the abdominal wall, usually near the belly button. The bladder can be emptied by passing a catheter through the stoma or a bag may be worn on the abdomen to collect the urine. From M. B. Chancellor & J. G. Blaivas, *Genitourinary Complications in Neurologic Disease*, *Practical Neuro-Urology*, Butterworth Heinemann, Boston, 1995, with permission.

cancer. In these people, the only available option is urinary diversion. There are two kinds of urinary diversions—urinary reservoirs and urinary conduits.

A urinary reservoir is constructed by isolating a segment of the intestine and reconfiguring it into the shape of a sphere that serves as a new bladder. One end of the sphere is connected to the ureters (the muscular tubes that drain urine from the kidneys), and another piece of intestine is reconfigured into the shape and function of the urethra and attached to another part of the sphere (Figure 2). This new urethra may be brought out to the skin of the abdominal wall or sewn in place to the remaining urethra. Depending on the circumstances, the patient either voids through this urethra or performs intermittent self-catheterization.

A urinary conduit provides drainage of urine to a small opening in the skin, called a stoma. Urine constantly drains through this stoma and is stored in a drainage bag that is applied directly to the skin. The bag is emptied of urine three or four times a day. The ileal loop, or Bricker operation, is the most commonly performed conduit (Figure 3).

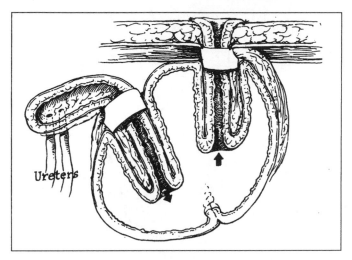

Figure 2. Urinary reservoir. A piece of intestine was disconnected from the remaining intestine and made into the shape of a sphere. Two nipples were created from either end of the intestine. One nipple was connected to the skin, forming a stoma. The other was connected to the ureters to drain urine from the kidneys. The arrows point to the direction of urine flow.

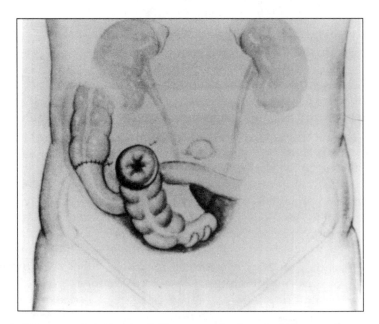

Figure 3. Urinary conduit (ileal loop). The two ureters from the kidney are shown attached to the short segment of intestine (the conduit). The other end of the intestine comes out to the skin. The puckered opening is called a stoma. Urine drains from the kidneys through the ureters, into the conduit, and out the stoma into a drainage bag on the skin (not pictured), where it is stored.

DESCRIPTION OF SURGERY

All of these operations are major surgeries that require an inpatient stay of about 3 to 10 days or more. Because your intestines will be used in the operation, preoperative bowel preparation is necessary. This means that all bowel contents (feces) need to be evacuated and the bowel sterilized. The bowel prep usually begins on the day prior to surgery. You'll probably be instructed to have a liquid diet and you'll be given a cathartic to clean out the intestinal tract. There are many different regimens for this, but the one I prefer is a preparation called Go-Litely. It is a drink that causes you to have diarrhea, which completely cleanses the bowel. In some patients, particularly those with spinal cord injury or spina bifida, enemas must be given as well. It may be necessary to administer intravenous fluids so that you don't become dehydrated. Several antibiotics must also be given in order to sterilize the bowel contents.

The operation is performed through an incision that extends from just below the rib cage in the midline to just above the pubic bone. The abdominal cavity is entered and a portion of the intestine is separated from the rest of the intestine (Figure 4). The remaining intestine is sutured back

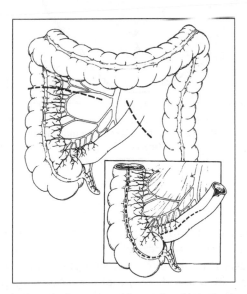

Figure 4. Isolating the intestinal segment. A long tube of intestine is removed from the rest of the intestine by cutting on the dotted lines.   (Inset) An incision is made along the whole length of the isolated segment of intestine (dotted line) converting it from the shape of a long tube to a rectangle. From R. Luangkhot, B. Peng, & J. G. Blaivas, "Ileocecocystoplasty for the Management of Refractory Neurogenic Bladder: Surgical Technique and Urodynamic Findings," *J. Urol.* 146:1340, 1991, with permission.

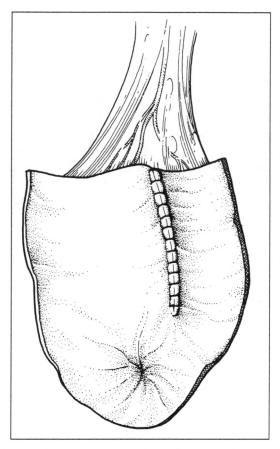

Figure 5. Reconfiguring the intestine into the shape of a sphere. The intestine is opened and folded into the shape of a half sphere and the sides of the intestine are sewn together. From R. Luangkhot, B. Peng, & J. G. Blaivas, "Ileocecocystoplasty for the Management of Refractory Neurogenic Bladder: Surgical Technique and Urodynamic Findings," *J. Urol.* 146:1340, 1991, with permission.

together. The detached intestine is opened with a scalpel along its entire length so that it is no longer a tube, but rather a long rectangle. If an augmentation cystoplasty is to be done, the rectangle of intestine is folded on itself and the edges sewn together so that it becomes shaped like half a sphere (Figure 5).

Next, the bladder is opened and also surgically reconfigured to form half of a sphere (Figure 6). The two spherical halves are sewn together (the intestinal segment on top, the bladder segment on the bottom). A catheter

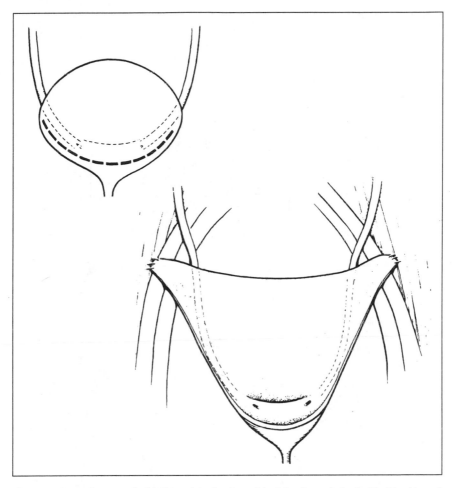

Figure 6. Reconfiguring the bladder. A smile-shaped incision is made in the bladder (dotted line) and it is sewn to the muscles on either side to hold it open. This converts it into the shape of half a sphere. From R. Luangkhot, B. Peng, & J. G. Blaivas, "Ileocecocystoplasty for the Management of Refractory Neurogenic Bladder: Surgical Technique and Urodynamic Findings," *J. Urol.* 146:1340, 1991, with permission.

(suprapubic tube) is left in the augmented bladder to drain the urine until the incisions heal (Figure 7).

If a urinary reservoir is to be done, the intestine is folded and sutured together to form a sphere, one end of which is connected to the ureters and the other end will be sutured to either the urethra or the skin as described above (see Figure 2).

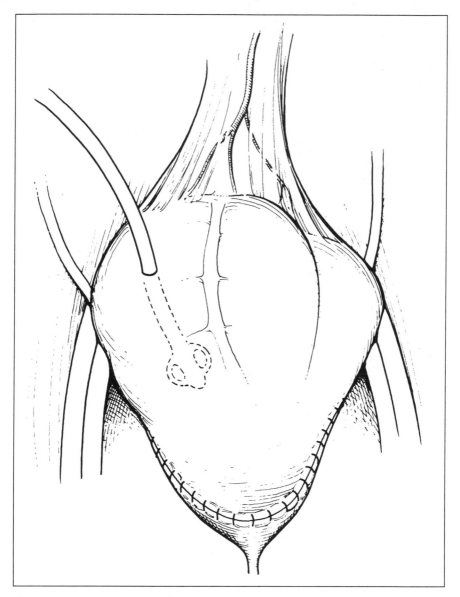

Figure 7. Formation of the augmentation cystoplasty. The two half-spheres (the reconfigured intestine on top and the reconfigured bladder on the bottom) are sutured together completing the augmentation. A catheter is inserted into the augmented bladder to drain urine until it heals. From R. Luangkhot, B. Peng, & J. G. Blaivas, "Ileocecocystoplasty for the Management of Refractory Neurogenic Bladder: Surgical Technique and Urodynamic Findings," *J. Urol.* 146:1340, 1991, with permission.

POSTOPERATIVE CARE

At the time of surgery, one or more catheters will be left in place in order to drain urine until everything heals. There will be at least one catheter to drain urine from the reservoir or augmented bladder. There may also be one or two tubes (stents) that go from each kidney through the ureter and come out the skin or stoma to drain urine directly from the kidneys. These are generally removed within the first 5–10 days after surgery. You will also probably have a drain (rubberlike tube) coming out of the abdomen to prevent infection. Some doctors also routinely use a nasogastric tube (a tube that is passed through your nose into your stomach) until the intestines are working OK. I don't think this is necessary and I don't use them. Of course, you will have an intravenous line for the administration of fluid and nourishment until the intestine begins to work and you can start to eat.

You should be out of bed and beginning to walk with some help on the day after surgery. Of course, there will be some pain, but it should be well controlled with pain medications. Thereafter, each day should be a little better than the day before. You will have nothing to eat until there are signs that the bowels are working. This usually takes about three days. Once you are feeling reasonably well, and able to eat OK, you may be discharged from the hospital, usually after four to five days, but some patients do not feel so well and may remain in the hospital for ten days or more.

POTENTIAL COMPLICATIONS

As with any other procedure there are potential complications. Life-threatening complications are very rare and occur in less than 1% of patients. Internal bleeding is a potential complication but, for practical purposes, it is very rare unless the operation is being done in conjunction with removal of the bladder for cancer. Respiratory (breathing) complications such as collapse of a portion of a lung or pneumonia are not uncommon in this or any other abdominal operation but are usually quite minor and rarely prolong the hospital stay. The usual treatment is physiotherapy to the lungs and sometimes antibiotics.

There is always a possibility of wound infection. This generally occurs on the seventh to fourteenth day and begins as a gradual increase in abdominal pain followed by tenderness and redness of the wound. Once the diagnosis is apparent, the wound needs to be surgically drained. This is usually accomplished by simply removing the sutures and opening the wound with a finger at the bedside. It is usually not painful to do this. Sometimes the wound spontaneously opens and begins to drain by itself. Complete disruption of the wound is a rare complication that is usually restricted to patients in poor health and particularly those with poor nutritional status. When this occurs, a secondary operation to close the wound must be performed. Obese patients or those with a history of previous urinary infections have a much higher likelihood of developing wound infection.

Urinary tract infections are occasionally seen during the immediate postoperative course and these are generally treated with antibiotics. A positive urine culture, however, is the rule after these operations and by itself does not necessarily indicate the presence of an infection.

The most serious complications are bowel obstruction, ureteral obstruction, and leakage of urine through the reservoir or conduit into the abdominal cavity. Bowel obstruction can occur if the intestine becomes scarred or twisted. The usual symptoms are nausea, vomiting, and crampy abdominal pain. It is generally treated by passing a nasogastric tube through the nose into the stomach and into the intestine to decompress the blockage. In some instances, a secondary operation is needed to relieve the obstruction.

Ureteral obstruction (a blockage of the ureter) is uncommon, and when it occurs, it usually is diagnosed years later. Occasionally a secondary operation is necessary to fix the obstruction. Urinary leakage into the abdominal cavity is very common immediately after surgery and generally of no consequence. Rarely, however, it can persist for many days or weeks. If this occurs, it is usually treated by passing a tube into the conduit or reservoir until it has healed. In rare instances, this may also require a secondary operation.

The possible long-term complications include bowel obstruction, recurrent infections, kidney stones, troublesome diarrhea, vitamin deficiency, and deterioration of the kidneys. There have been a few very rare reports of the development of cancer in the augmented bladder, but this does not appear to be any more common than if you never had the operation in the first place. In general, the chances of these latter complications are far less after this surgery than they would have been if the bladder condition was left the way it was. Further, as a general rule, the most important complications—deterioration of the kidney, kidney stones, and infection—are much more common after conduits than after reservoirs or augmentation cystoplasty.

Those sound like very serious complications. Why would I ever choose a urinary conduit? So how do I decide between a reservoir and a conduit?

The decision is not an easy one. All of the theoretical considerations strongly favor the construction of a reservoir or continent diversion. Ideally you would remain perfectly dry and do self intermittent catheterization only three or four times a day. You need not wear an appliance and the site of the stoma can be placed inconspicuously enough that no one need know you even have one. Most often I put it in the belly button where it can't be seen at all. You can go into a regular stall or bathroom and catheterize yourself without anyone knowing. Because the physiology of the reservoir is similar to that of the bladder (it accommodates to very large volumes of urine at very low bladder pressure), the chances of developing kidney deterioration are remote.

On the other hand, construction of a reservoir is a time-consuming and technically demanding procedure that only a few surgeons have mastered. The procedure has only recently gained any degree of popularity; accordingly, there are no meaningful long-term studies of the effects of continent urinary diversion. In addition, the surgical techniques are still in a state of evolution. Construction of the reservoir is straightforward and has few complications. On the other hand, construction of the valve mechanism to prevent urine from leaking out through the stoma is a much more demanding and as yet unperfected procedure, and some people will need to undergo secondary operations to repair malfunctions in this valve mechanism or stoma.

Construction of the urinary conduit is a much simpler operation, although it is still a major surgery that does add inherent risks to the kidneys that are lacking in the continent urinary diversion. The incidence of kidney stones, infection, and damage to the kidneys is likely to be much higher after a conduit than after a reservoir or augmentation cystoplasty. Nevertheless, it is still quite safe and certainly safer than the other usual options such as being treated with an indwelling bladder catheter continuously. Most people will not choose a urinary conduit if they have the option of a reservoir. However, all of the complications that I just alluded to are amenable to early diagnosis, prevention, and treatment provided that you return for annual surveillance. Severe complications, for practical purposes, only occur in patients who do not receive proper follow-up. If you have an otherwise unmanageable problem with incontinence and you are not a candidate for urinary reservoir, a urinary conduit or an ileal chimney is a most reasonable choice. If I had such a problem, I'd probably have an ileal chimney.

CONCLUSION

Rarely, the bladder or the urethra is so severely damaged that it no longer serves its intended purpose and the person is rendered hopelessly incontinent. No matter how severe the damage, it is still possible for a person to achieve complete continence, remain confidently dry, and lead a normal life after reconstructive surgery. Reconstructive operations, which use part of the intestines to replace the functions of the bladder and urethra, are of two kinds: one is called cystoplasty; the other, urinary diversion. Cystoplasty makes the bladder much bigger and able to hold larger amounts of urine so that the patient can remain confidently dry. However, most patients cannot urinate well and need to empty their bladder with intermittent self-catheterization that needs to be done three or four times a day.

There are two kinds of urinary diversions—conduits and reservoirs. Urinary conduits completely bypass the bladder. Instead of being stored in the bladder, urine is stored in an external appliance—a drainage bag on the abdomen—that is emptied periodically throughout the day. The conduit is made from a segment of intestine that bridges the gap between the ureters (to which it is attached on one end) and the skin of the abdomen (the stoma). Urine flows from the kidneys through the ureters, through the conduit, and out through the stoma into the drainage bag, where the urine is stored.

Urinary reservoirs replace the function of the bladder. They are also made from a segment of intestine that is reconfigured into the shape of a sphere. The ureters are attached to one end and the other end is either sutured to the urethra or fashioned into an abdominal stoma. If an abdominal stoma is used, it needs to be emptied by intermittent catheterization. If the reservoir is attached to the urethra, it may be possible to urinate naturally, but most people still need intermittent catheterization.

21

Absorbent Pads, Appliances, and Other Products for Controlling Incontinence

INTRODUCTION

The goal of any therapy for incontinence is to restore normal urination and to avoid the use of indwelling catheters, pads, or appliances, While this is a realistic goal and can be obtained for the majority of patients, there are some for whom perfect urinary control is either not possible or not desirable.

Why would a person prefer to remain incontinent and use diapers or pads?

I don't think anyone prefers to be incontinent. No one prefers pads or diapers, but many patients have mild enough degrees of incontinence that they really don't want to undergo surgery, take medications, or undergo intensive behavioral modification programs for a problem that they consider to be mild and to which they've grown accustomed.

If you have incontinence that is not completely controlled, for whatever reason, there are a number of different methods available for keeping you confidently dry. For mild degrees of incontinence, a piece of absorbent toilet tissue or paper towel placed in your underwear as a liner may suffice. Unfortunately, many people use this method, even if it doesn't suffice. They stuff their underwear with tissues and towels in a desperate attempt at staying dry, but the amount of urinary loss cannot be controlled by this method. Out of ignorance (with a little help from unsympathetic insurance companies and some health care professionals), they think that nothing else can be done and they simply give up and do the best they can, changing their clothes frequently throughout the day. Some become social outcasts because wherever they go, the odor of urine is ever present. Others simply never leave home and lead lives of lonely isolation. The pity of it all is that, even for people whose incontinence cannot be cured or treated, there are ample methods for managing the urinary loss. That means that, no matter how bad or uncontrollable the incontinence is, there are products that you can use which will either absorb the urine or divert it into a collection device so that your underwear or clothes will not get wet. There will be no odors, and no one will know you have the problem unless you choose to tell them.

The main problem, though, is that not very many people know about these products. Most doctors, even urologists and gynecologists, don't know about these things. Most nurses don't either. But some do, and if you are having difficulty managing incontinence, it would be best to seek them out. If your doctor has not been helpful in this regard and no one in his office is helpful either, the chances are that somewhere in your community there is an ostomy nurse; if you're lucky there is a continence advisor. An ostomy nurse is a specially trained person who helps patients (and their doctors) care for ostomies. An ostomy is a small opening in the abdomen intentionally made during an operation to connect an organ such as the intestine or urinary tract to the skin. These operations are usually performed after a part of the intestine or urinary tract has been removed for cancer, but they are also occasionally done for patients with otherwise unmanageable incontinence. I call an ostomy a stoma and so do most of the people that I talk to. The stoma, then, is nothing more than a hole in the abdomen connected to the intestine or urinary tract surgically created in order to manage a difficult problem of eliminating stool or urine. Figure 1 shows a drawing of a stoma.

There are two ways of managing the stoma—with an appliance or with intermittent catheterization. An appliance is a collection device that is placed around the stoma, secured with an adhesive, into which the urine or stool flows through the stoma. It is also possible for the surgeon to construct the stoma so that it acts as a valve to prevent urinary leakage, but the person has to drain the urine with a catheter periodically throughout the day. An ostomy nurse is someone who is expert in all of the different kinds of problems that a person with an ostomy (stoma) experiences. A continence advisor is a specially trained health care professional, usually a nurse, who is expert on many different ways to manage incontinence, including intermittent catheterization and the use of pads and appliances.

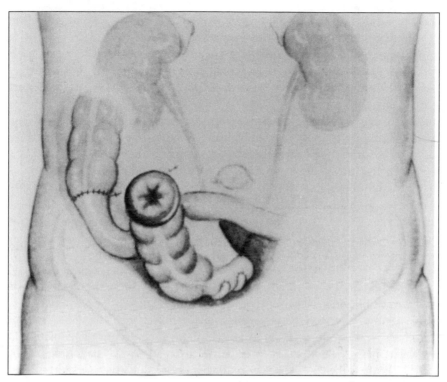

Figure 1. Urinary conduit (ileal loop). The two ureters from the kidney are shown attached to a short segment of intestine (the conduit). The other end of the intestine comes out to the skin. The puckered opening is called a stoma. Urine drains from the kidneys through the ureters, into the conduit, and out the stoma into a drainage bag on the skin (not pictured), where it is stored.

Whether or not you can find a competent ostomy nurse or continence advisor, there are many commonsense ways of managing the problem of incontinence. The most ubiquitous method is the use of absorbent pads. There are also a number of brand-new products on the market that attempt to block the urethra using adhesive materials applied directly to the meatus (the outside opening of the urethra) so that urine simply can't get out of the body. There are new urethral inserts, little tubes that go into the urethra blocking the flow of urine. These must be removed each time you urinate. There is even a new device that has a magnetically operated valve that can be opened and closed each time you want to urinate. For men, there are a number of condom catheter devices. These are plastic or elastic materials that are placed around the penis as a sheath. Although there has been much previous and ongoing research to offer a similar collection device to women, none has been very effective.

For patients who are unable to urinate at all or don't empty their bladders completely enough, there are only two currently available options—intermittent catheterization and an indwelling bladder catheter. However, at present there is a considerable amount of research in this area and there are several ingenious devices currently being investigated. The most promising of these is a small catheter with a valve to keep you dry and a little turbine that actually propels the urine out of your bladder into the toilet just like normal urination. It is currently undergoing clinical trials in the United States, but there is not yet enough information available for me to judge whether it is safe or effective. I hope it works!

ABSORBENT PADS

The sale of absorbent pads to manage urinary incontinence is reportedly a multibillion dollar industry. Why would that be? There are two possible reasons. First, too many people, sadly, still have the mistaken notion that there isn't very much that can be done for incontinence and that pads are about all they can do to keep themselves dry. If you've gotten this far in this book, though, you probably realize by now that that is not at all the case. Second, people do not consider their incontinence to be enough of a problem to warrant further treatment, because the pads work just fine.

No matter what the reasons, absorbent pads are probably still the most common form of treatment for people with urinary incontinence. Pads come in a wide assortment of sizes and types. They range from mini-pads and panty liners to adult diapers. The former can generally hold 5 to 10 oz. and prevent leakage to your outer clothing; the latter can hold 100 ozs. or more.

EXTERNAL URINARY DEVICES FOR MEN

Among other things, a penis is good for holding appliances to drain urine if you are incontinent. One kind of appliance for this purpose is called a condom catheter. A condom catheter looks like an ordinary condom, but it has a hole in the end near the tip of the penis (I don't recommend that you use this for contraception). The condom is pulled over the penis to which it is attached with an adhesive or a strap. At the tip of the catheter where the hole is, there is a tube that connects to a drainage bag, which is worn on the leg. Urine flows through the condom, through the tube, and into the bag, which is emptied periodically. Condom catheters are most often used in patients with neurologic disorders but occasionally may be used in men with severe sphincteric incontinence. If the condom catheter is applied too tightly, which is particularly a problem if there is a neurologic disease that impairs sensation, it can cause irritation and even severe infection or gangrene of the penis. Another complication of condom catheters, particularly in neurologic patients, is a blockage to the flow of urine. The pressure builds up in the urethra behind the blockage and a diverticulum, or outpouching, of the urethra can occur. Accordingly, the condom should be checked periodically throughout the day to be sure that it is not too tight, and the condom should be changed daily.

Another type of appliance for men is a small pouch made of an absorbent material that goes around the penis, but is not secured to it. When urine leaks out, it is absorbed by the pouch, which is discarded periodically throughout the day.

EXTERNAL DEVICES FOR WOMEN

Given that women do not have a penis that can hold a collection device, it takes more imagination to devise a suitable appliance. At the present time, there are a number of commercially available products that claim to work well, but none works nearly as well as I would like. Maybe by the time this book is finally published, things will be better. Maybe not. If you use pads or diapers, you can experiment and improvise, but you can't do that very well with the external devices for women. They either work or they don't. There are two general kinds of devices of which I am aware—adhesive patches and urethral inserts. An adhesive patch, made of a soft, plastic material, is placed over the urethral opening (meatus) to block the urine from leaking out. Some products are little more than a piece of clear plastic tape. A urethral insert, or stent, is a small tube that is inserted into the urethra to block the flow of urine. It is usually held in place either by a little balloon inside the bladder or by a flange that collapses as the stent is pulled out. The problem with most of these devices is that they have to be changed or reinserted each time you urinate. That can be expensive and uncomfortable. Also, if they are not changed often enough they can cause urinary tract infection and even stones. Further, the long-term consequences of these devices are unknown. Other products being tested are actually urethral stents with miniature valves inside. They stay in place in the urethra for about a month at a time. The valve is supposed to keep urine from leaking out, like a sphincter. It is opened with a magnetic or battery-operated hand-held activator when you want to urinate. When you're done urinating, you close the valve with the activator.

PESSARIES AND BLADDER NECK PROSTHESES

A pessary is an appliance, like a diaphragm, which is placed in the vagina to hold a prolapsed organ in place. They are usually shaped like a donut and come in many different sizes. Many people with prolapse have bladder symptoms. Sometimes the dropped bladder actually causes a blockage and you're either unable to urinate at all, or you have difficulty urinating. If you push or strain, that only makes the prolapse worse and it becomes even harder to void. In other people, the prolapse causes discomfort, aching, or a constant feeling that you have to urinate. In some people, the bladder becomes hypersensitive or overactive and you have to urinate very frequently. If you have any of these symptoms and you have a dropped bladder, uterus, or rectum, a pessary may relieve all of your symptoms. Pessaries come in many different sizes and shapes. Your doctor will choose the one that is most appropriate for you and decide on the proper fit. Unfortunately, there is no simple way to attain the proper fit or choose the best kind of pessary. It's all trial and error. Your doctor will examine you and try a certain type or size. Then, if it feels comfortable, you should get up and walk around and see how it feels. If it is comfortable and stays in place, and relieves your symptoms, you may prefer the pessary to other forms of treatment. Further, some pessaries are shaped so that they also hold the sphincter in place and can be used to treat stress incontinence. These are called bladder neck prostheses. They've only been available for a year or two, so there isn't any meaningful data about how effective they are. But they do work in some people and they do not to my knowledge do any serious harm. Of course, any pessary or bladder neck prosthesis can cause inflammation, infection, or even an erosion of the vaginal wall, so they need to be checked by your doctor periodically. If you do not have any particular infirmities, you probably will be able to insert and remove the pessary yourself. Many people use the pessary only when they are going out or exercising or whenever else they think it is necessary. Even if you can't put it in and take it out yourself, you can use a pessary if you want to. Your doctor can fit you, insert it, then remove it at three-month intervals, wash it off, inspect the vagina, and put it back in, provided that there are no vaginal erosions or infections.

How do I know if a pessary would be a good idea for me?

The only way to know if a pessary is for you is to try it. You might like it. But follow the instructions carefully.

SKIN CARE AND DEODORIZING PRODUCTS

Believe it or not, most of the time, normal urine does not have an odor and, in small volumes, does not irritate your skin. However, sometimes normal urine does have an offensive odor and, in some people, it may be very irritating to the skin. No matter what, though, if urine is allowed to remain on clothing, pads, or appliances, bacteria will grow and their waste products do have an offensive odor and they do irritate the skin. So the best way to prevent odor and to be kind to your skin is to be sure that you change your pads frequently.

How frequently should I change them?

As a general rule you should change whenever they seem more than damp or moist. When in doubt, let your nose or your skin be your guide. No matter how often you change, though, there may be an offensive odor or your skin may become irritated. Fortunately, if this happens to you there are many effective deodorizing sprays and tablets and there are many skin care products.

INTERMITTENT CATHETERIZATION

Over the last two or three decades, intermittent catheterization has proven to be the single most important advance in the treatment of patients with refractory bladder problems causing either incontinence or inability to urinate. Intermittent catheterization may be used as a temporary means of managing your bladder while you are awaiting other therapies, or it may be used as definitive treatment over a lifetime. Except in the most unusual of circumstances, you should do intermittent catheterization yourself and not rely on a nurse, aide, or family member. If you do the catheterization yourself, it is called self intermittent catheterization (SIC). SIC is generally meant to replace normal urination, but sometimes, particularly if you are unable to urinate after surgery, you should try to urinate first, then catheterize yourself. Most authorities agree that when doing SIC, there is no need for sterile tech-

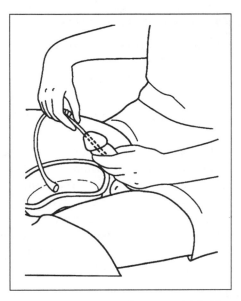

Figure 2. Self intermittent catheterization in a man. From M. B. Chancellor & J. G. Blaivas, *Genitourinary Complication in Neurologic Disease, Practical Neuro-Urology,* Butterworth-Heinemann, Boston, 1995, with permission.

nique; there is no need for gloves; there is no need for antiseptic solutions. All that is necessary is a catheter and some lubrication to allow easy insertion of the catheter into the urethra. The procedure is simple. You go into a bathroom, sit or stand, put a dab of lubricant on the tip of the catheter and insert the catheter into the penis and through the urethra into the bladder in men (Figure 2) and into the vaginal opening of the urethra in women (Figure 3). Once the catheter is inside the bladder, urine will begin to flow out and you should keep the catheter in place until the urine stops flowing. You may assist the urine flow by pushing down on your abdomen; this will cause the urine to come out faster. In general, within the limits of comfort, the larger the size of the catheter the easier it is to insert and the faster the urine comes out. For that reason relatively larger sizes (16–18 french) are more desirable than smaller catheters (8–14 french).

In addition to being used for permanent management of a urinary problem, intermittent catheterization is very useful in patients for whom complete recovery is expected but has not yet occurred. This most commonly is the situation immediately after many different kinds of surgeries. Some patients after surgery, for whatever reason, are unable to urinate at

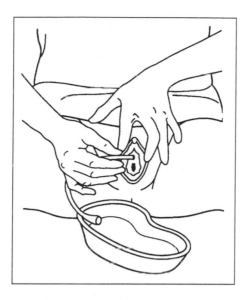

Figure 3. Self intermittent catheterization in a woman. From M. B. Chancellor & J. G. Blaivas, *Genitourinary Complication in Neurologic Disease, Practical Neuro-Urology,* Butterworth-Heinemann, Boston, 1995, with permission.

all. Traditionally, this has been managed by leaving an indwelling catheter in place, then removing the catheter when the doctor thinks that the patient ought to be able to void. Then, the patient would undergo a "voiding trial." This means that after the catheter is removed, you wait until urine builds up in your bladder and you have the urge to urinate. You're then, for practical purposes, given one chance to urinate and if you can't go, the catheter goes back in place for another several days. You can imagine the emotional and psychological trauma that accompanies this kind of treatment. It's almost like a punishment: You're given one chance to urinate and if you can't, back goes the catheter! This causes an incredible amount of pressure on the patient to urinate, and under these circumstances he or she is very often unable to do so. Intermittent self-catheterization completely avoids this problem. Using this technique you wait until you get the urge to urinate, you go into the bathroom, and try. Whether or not your urinate, you then catheterize yourself. When the residual volumes of urine are low enough catheterization can be discontinued. There is no psychological pressure to void because you know that you are in control and that you won't have to walk around day to day with an indwelling catheter and then get only one chance to urinate once it's removed.

I don't want to do intermittent self-cauterization and I don't want anybody else to catheterize me four times per day. I could never learn to do that! This all sounds barbaric!

Nearly everyone can learn to do intermittent catheterization. It is painless and not at all uncomfortable. For the vast majority of people who need to do intermittent catheterization, rather than being barbaric or a nuisance, it has been a godsend. It is the closest thing to normal urination that you can obtain. If you can't urinate at all, there really isn't any other alternative except for an indwelling catheter. If you're hopelessly incontinent or in the bathroom twenty times a day urinating or changing pads and diapers, with self-catheterization you are now in the bathroom three, four, or five times a day and you're confidently dry.

What about infection? I would think that with all that catheterization there must be a terrible problem with urinary infection.

Quite to the contrary. Most patients that have the kinds of problems that require intermittent catheterization are already at considerable risk for developing urinary tract infections and most have had infections in the past. Although intermittent catheterization doesn't insure against infections, the chances of developing infection are much, much less with intermittent catheterization than with either the way you're urinating now or any other treatment method.

History of Intermittent Catheterization

Believe it or not, urethral catheterization has been used for over 3000 years. The Sushruta Samhita, an early Indian surgical text written in approximately 1000 B.C., described catheters that were made of gold, silver, iron, and even wood. They were smeared with ghee (a kind of liquid butter) and passed into the urethra, not only to empty the bladder but also for stretching (dilating) urethral scars (strictures) and even for removing stones from the bladder. (1,2) Sushruta suggested that "wine should be used before operation to produce insensibility to pain." Can you imagine that! Before anesthesia! Before sterility! Before antibiotics! Hippocrates (460 to 37 B.C.) wrote about catheters and removing stones. By tradition, the Hippocratic Oath is taken by all physicians upon their graduation from medical school. Part of that oath is to pledge that only urologists should remove stones from the bladder. Of course, there wasn't any such thing as a urologist back then, but there were lithotomists. Lithotomy literally means "cutting for stone." A lithotomist was a doctor trained to "cut for stone." Hippocrates was apparently the first to recognize the need for specialists in medicine. (3)

For practical purposes, though, intermittent catheterization was almost never used until the pioneering work of two doctors named Guttmann and Frankel, who began to experiment with its use in the management of people with neurogenic bladder during the 1950s. Guttmann, one of the first specialists in spinal cord injury, recognized the dangers of bladder overstretching and realized the importance of proper draining of the bladder and that it was mandatory to the survival of people with spinal cord injury. (4) He also realized that an indwelling catheter did not at all prevent infection or stones or the inevitable progression to kidney failure. He began to have his spinal cord injury patients treated with intermittent catheterization by the nursing staff, and the results were impressive. A fixed catheterization time schedule (approximately every four to eight hours) was used. (5) However, this method of treatment was very expensive, time consuming, and required so much equipment (catheters, gloves, drapes, irrigation catheters, bottles of fluid) that you would need a small truck to leave the hospital or your home if you used a sterile technique. Even if sterile technique was important, it was too impractical.

It was Jack Lapides, former Professor and Chairman of Urology at the University of Michigan (6), who really introduced and popularized the use of clean (nonsterile) intermittent catheterization. Dr. Lapides was convinced that it was elevated bladder pressure and stasis of urine from incomplete bladder emptying that caused the serious kidney infections and stones that ultimately caused kidney failure and death in more than half of spinal cord injury patients. He believed that these two factors—bladder pressure and stasis of urine—were more important than the bacteria itself, a revolutionary thought at the time. The first clean SIC patient was a woman with neurogenic bladder due to multiple sclerosis who had been getting repeated infections with an indwelling bladder catheter. At first, she was taught SIC with sterile technique. She did so well that it changed her life around. She became continent, free of infection, and traveled to Europe. While there, she dropped her sterile catheter on the floor of a public bathroom, and, unable to resterilize it, she simply proceeded with her catheterization with no ill effect. (7) In 1971, Dr. Lapides presented a paper on this approach to the prestigious American Association of Genito-Urinary Surgeons, stating that "Intermittent catheterization of the bladder should be an innocuous procedure provided the bladder is not permitted to overdistend and a clean and not aseptic technique should suffice since any bacteria introduced by the catheter will be neutralized by the resistance of the host." (8) The ensuing decades have proved him right in many if not in most cases.

INDWELLING CATHETERS

For the urologist, indwelling catheters are to be avoided at all costs. They cause infection, they cause kidney damage, they can erode through the urethra, causing incontinence, and they can cause bladder and kidney stones. In men, they cause strictures, or scars, in the urethra that, after removal of the catheter, can cause serious blockages, and rarely, they can cause bladder or urethral cancer. For the patient, particularly women who cannot catheterize themselves either because of disability or infirmity due to age, there may be no other practical solution.

Those sound like awful complications; why would anyone use an indwellng catheter?

Well, as I alluded to above, for some patients there simply isn't any other alternative. In addition, short-term catheter use—that is, for days, weeks, or a few months—is very unlikely to cause any of those problems. Further, the chances of those complications occurring, even with long-term catheter use, can be greatly minimized if a number of precautions are taken. First, within the limitations of comfort, the larger the catheter you use, the better and safer.

Why would a large catheter be preferable to a smaller one?

A large catheter has a larger hole that is less likely to become twisted or blocked and the flow of urine through the catheter is much more likely to be unimpeded. Small catheters actually are smaller than the natural urethra. This means that every time the bladder contracts it is as if there is a blockage; in fact, there is a blockage—the catheter itself. The long-term consequences of blockages in the urethra are bladder damage, kidney damage, stones, infections, etc., and for all of these reasons a larger rather than a smaller catheter is preferable.

But doesn't the large catheter hurt more than the small catheter?

In fact, no. It's only if the catheter gets so large that it stretches the urethra that it might be painful. The catheter sizes that we're talking about are all small enough to be comfortable for the great majority of patients. Further, a larger catheter is easier to pass into the urethra because it is stiffer than a small catheter.

The second precaution to take is to change the catheter as often as is practical. Under no circumstances should the same catheter be left in place for more than about a month, but it is far preferable to change it at weekly or biweekly intervals. The longer the same catheter stays in the bladder, the greater the chances of the bladder developing incrustations, blockages, and stone formation.

CONCLUSION

For patients with urinary incontinence or difficulty urinating, the goal of treatment is to restore normal functioning, but this is not always possible. Further, for some people, the symptoms themselves are of so little concern that they prefer the use of pads or appliances to manage their problem. Fortunately, modern technology has advanced to the point where nearly every person can be managed to his or her own level of satisfaction. For some, this means surgery or medications. For others, pads and appliances are just fine. For still others, intermittent self-catheterization is what works best.

You've just mentioned an awful lot of options. How will I ever choose?

The best advice I can give is trial and error particularly under the guidance of a knowledgeable and highly trained physician or nurse. If you are lucky, your local pharmacy carries enough incontinence products for you to experiment with; if not, complain to the pharmacy that they don't carry enough products and get the resource guide from the National Association for Continence (NAFC). This guide has a description and picture of almost every imaginable product. The resource guide is published annually by the National Association for Continence. The address is listed in Appendix B. This resource guide lists over 1000 products for managing incontinence placed into 12 categories, including disposable and reusable absorbent pads and diapers; external urinary devices such as condom catheters, penile clamps, and pouches for men; urethral plugs, inserts, and patches for women. They also list leg bags and other devices for storing urine and skin care and deodorizing products.

NOTES

1. Das, S., Shusruta of India, the pioneer in the treatment of urethral stricture. *Surg. Gynec. Bost.* 157 (1983):581.

2. Bloom, D. A., McGuire, E. J., & Lapides, J., A brief history of urethral catheterization. *J. Urol.* 151 (1994):317–325.
3. Adams, F., *The Genuine Works of Hippocrates.* London, UK: Sydenham Society, 1849, 736–779.
4. Bloom et al., A brief history.
5. Guttmann, L., & Frankel, H., The value of intermittent catheterization in the early management of traumatic paraplegia and tetraplegia. *Paraplegia* 4 (1966):63.
6. Lapides, J., Diokno, A. C., & Silber, S. J., Clean intermittent self-catherization in the treatment of urinary tract disease. *J. Urol.* 107 (1972):458.
7. Bloom et al., A brief history.
8. Lapides, J., Diokno, A. C., Silber, S. J., & Lowe, B. S., Clean intermittent self-catheterization in the treatment of urinary tract disease. *Trans. Am. Ass. Genito-Urinary Surg.* 63 (1971):92.

Epilogue

The message of this book is a simple one. Bladder and prostate problems cause symptoms that, in the majority of people, are diagnosable and treatable, and for most, even curable—provided that you are treated by a competent physician. Armed with the knowledge that I've tried to impart, you should be able to find a competent physician, because you've learned how your body works and what can go wrong and how to fix it. You've learned what the doctor should do and what to expect. You should expect to get better.

A word of warning. There are two approaches to medicine, a statistical approach and an individualized approach. Both are based on what I call degrees of certainty. Degrees of certainty refer to the probability of your doctor diagnosing your condition correctly and recommending a treatment that is likely to work. For example, if you have blood in your urine, you probably have a urinary tract infection and you'll probably get better with antibiotics. Your doctor will treat you with antibiotics and if you don't get better, he will try another antibiotic. That's the statistical approach and it works for most people. But if you have blood in your urine, you may have bladder cancer, not an infection. So, alternatively, your doctor orders a urinalysis, a culture, and sensitivities. If it shows infection, he treats you with antibiotics; if not, he orders certain tests and exams to check for cancer. If you do have cancer, you get early diagnosis and treatment. That's the individualized approach.

Most of the time the statistical approach works, and even when it doesn't, you eventually get the right diagnosis, because the proper tests are eventually done. Usually you even get the right treatment (albeit a little late) and most of the time you're cured anyway. But not always.

The statistical approach is much less expensive than the individualized approach. Which approach you take depends on a number of things. It depends on your own and your doctor's comfort level with the degree of certainty of the diagnosis and proposed treatment, and it depends on who is paying the bill.

Glossary

Accommodation   A special property of the bladder wall that allows it to fill with urine at very low pressure. When you fill a balloon with air, the more the balloon increases in size, the greater the pressure inside the balloon and the harder you have to blow. This is because the walls of the balloon are made of a substance with elastic properties. Not so with the bladder. The bladder is composed of smooth muscle, collagen, and a small amount of elastic fibers (called elastin). When the bladder fills, its walls begin to stretch, but the bladder muscle (detrusor) relaxes. The net result is that the pressure in the bladder does not rise.

Acetylcholine   The chemical messenger (a neurotransmitter) that stimulates the bladder to contract.

Antibiotics   Substances that inhibit the growth of or kill microorganisms (bacteria and viruses). They are used to treat infections due to microorganisms.

Anticholinergic   A medication that blocks the action of acetylcholine. Anticholinergic medications are used to stop involuntary bladder contractions.

Antidiuretic hormone (ADH)   A substance produced by the pituitary gland in the brain. It signals the kidneys to cut back on urine production. It is normally secreted in response to dehydration.

Augmentation cystoplasty   An operation designed to increase the size of the bladder and stop the bladder from causing incontinence by contracting involuntarily. After augmentation cystoplasty, in many people the bladder can no longer empty itself and the person needs to perform intermittent catheterization.

Behavior modification   A method of treatment that is used for many conditions including interstitial cystitis, incontinence, and other painful blad-

der and prostate syndromes. It deals with observable and measurable behaviors that actually cause your symptoms and teaches you to change
those behaviors so that you no longer have those symptoms.

Bladder   The hollow, muscular organ that stores urine. It is composed of
a muscular component (detrusor) and a matrix between the muscle
fibers that is composed of many different tissues, including collagen,
elastin, and blood vessels.

Bladder compliance   A measure of bladder stiffness calculated by measuring the change in bladder volume over the change in bladder pressure. Normally as the bladder fills with urine, bladder pressure remains
very low despite very large changes in bladder volume. This results in
high bladder compliance, which is normal. In patients with low bladder
compliance, the bladder pressure rises considerably with small incre-
ments of bladder volume. This rise in pressure may overcome the resistance offered by the urethra and cause incontinence, or, if the sphincter
is strong or there is a urethral blockage, the high pressure is transmitted
back to the kidneys and ureters where it causes considerable damage
from back pressure.

BUN   An abbreviation for blood urea nitrogen, a blood test that measures how well the kidneys are working. Normal values are up to about
20 mg/dl. Values above this may mean that the kidneys are not working normally or that there is dehydration.

Catheter   A small rubber, latex, or silastic tube that is passed into the
bladder to drain the urine. A catheter may be stay in continuously (an
indwelling catheter) or be used for intermittent catheterization. See
Foley catheter and *suprapubic catheter.*

Condom catheter   A device used to collect urine and prevent incontinence in men. It is a silastic or rubber condom that goes around the
penis and is held in place with adhesive or Velcro. The tip of the condom is attached to tubing that goes to a drainage bag, usually worn on
the leg. Urine is directed by the condom through the tubing and into the
drainage bag, which needs to be emptied periodically throughout the
day.

Creatinine   A chemical in the bloodstream that is a measure of kidney
function. The upper limit of normal for most laboratories is 1.5 mg/dl.
Values above this mean that the kidneys are not working normally.

Culture-specific antibiotic   Antibiotics that prevent the growth of certain bacteria in a laboratory test. If bacterial growth is inhibited by a certain antibiotic, the bacteria are said to be sensitive to that antibiotic; if
not, they are said to be resistant to the antibiotic. To test whether or not
a particular antibiotic is effective, a drop of urine is "planted" on a cul-

ture plate containing agar, a jellylike substance full of nutrients that promote the growth and multiplication of bacteria. If there are bacteria in the urine, they will start to grow on the agar and, within a few days, they'll be visible to the naked eye. Scattered throughout the agar are little discs impregnated with different antibiotics. If the bacteria grow over a disc, the bacteria are resistant to that antibiotic. If there is a clear region of no bacterial growth around a disc, then the bacteria are sensitive to that antibiotic.

Cystocele A prolapse, or falling down, of the bladder into the vagina. It is commonly called a "dropped bladder."

Cystoplasty See *augmentation cystoplasty.*

Cystoscopy (Cystourethroscopy) A diagnostic examination performed by passing a thin telescopelike instrument (cystoscope) through the urethra into the bladder for the purpose of looking inside the bladder and urethra.

Detrusor The muscular component of the bladder wall.

Detrusor hyperreflexia Involuntary detrusor contractions caused by known neurologic conditions such as stroke, multiple sclerosis, spinal cord injury, and Parkinson's disease.

Detrusor instability Involuntary detrusor contractions that are not caused by known neurologic conditions. Detrusor instability is often associated with benign prostatic hyperplasia (enlargement of the prostate) and stress incontinence, but it is also often idiopathic.

Detrusor overactivity Involuntary bladder contractions. Involuntary detrusor contractions may cause a sensation of urgency or incontinence. There are two kinds of detrusor overactivity: detrusor hyperreflexia and detrusor instability.

Enterocele A prolapse, or falling down, of the intestines into the vagina.

FDA (Federal Drug Agency) The government agency that approves medications and medical devices for sale in the United States. FDA approval means that the FDA has sanctioned the safety and, to a lesser extent, the efficacy of a particular medication or device. FDA approval does *not* necessarily mean that the drug or device is effective, just that it might work and that it is probably safe. If a drug or device is approved for one condition and not for another, it doesn't mean that it is not safe or efficacious for the latter condition. If your doctor recommends that you use something that is not FDA approved for that use, it probably means that the company that makes or sells it didn't think it was worth the time and expense to get it approved for the use you are putting it to. In fact, for years, the most commonly prescribed medications for incontinence and prostate conditions were not approved for either use.

Fistula   An abnormal passage or connection between a hollow body cavity or organ and the surface of the body. See *vesicovaginal fistula* and *urethrovaginal fistula*.

Foley catheter   A catheter held in place with a little fluid-filled balloon at its end.

General anesthesia   A method of anesthesia that results in loss of sensation to your entire body to permit surgery or other painful procedures.

Gross hematuria   Blood in the urine that is visible to the naked eye, appearing in various shades of red.

Gynecologist   A physician and surgeon who specializes in the female reproductive and lower urinary tract.

Hematuria   Blood in the urine. See *microhematuria* and *gross hematuria*.

Idiopathic   Occurring without known cause.

Intermittent catheterization   Intermittent catheterization is a means of emptying the bladder when you cannot urinate normally. It may be used as a temporary method while you are awaiting or undergoing treatment, or it may be part of a permanent treatment program. Intermittent catheterization is performed by passing a catheter into the bladder (usually through the urethra) to empty the urine. It is usually done three to six times a day, depending on how much urine the bladder can safely hold. Intermittent catheterization done by the patient is called self intermittent catheterization (SIC).

Kidney   Two paired urine-making organs that lie in the small of your back, beneath the ribs and behind the abdomen. Their principal function is to filter liquid wastes and extra water from the bloodstream.

Lower urinary tract   The lower urinary tract consists of the bladder, prostate (in men), urethra, and urinary sphincter.

LUTS   Abbreviation for lower urinary tract symptoms; a group of symptoms that consist of (1) weak stream, (2) hesitancy (a delay before urination starts), (3) intermittency (an interrupted urinary stream), (4) frequency of urination, (5) urgency of urination (a feeling that you must rush to the bathroom or you might urinate without control, (6) nocturia (being awakened at night because of the need to urinate), (7) urge incontinence (loss of urinary control because of a strong urge to urinate), and (8) postvoid dribbling (a dribbling loss of urine that occurs immediately after urination).

Metastasis   The spread of cancer from the tissues in which it arose (primary cancer), to another part of the body. The most common site of spread is to adjacent lymph nodes, then to liver, lungs, or bone.

Microhematuria   Blood in the urine visible only under the microscope. Normally there are up to two red blood cells per high-powered field visible under the microscope. A greater number than this is considered to be microhematuria.

Micturition   Urination.

Monitored anesthesia care (MAC)   A method of providing anesthesia for short periods of time without the need for full general or regional anesthesia. It may be done as an adjunct to local anesthesia for procedures such as cystoscopy or bladder or prostate biopsy. It is scheduled with the attendance of an anesthesiologist, who can administer anesthesia if it is necessary. Usually an intravenous line is started and, depending on the degree of discomfort that you experience, the anesthesiologist can administer pain medication through the intravenous line or, if necessary, give you a general anesthesia to put you to sleep for the examination if the pain is too intense.

Necrosis   Death of individual cells or part of an organ.

Neonatal   The period of time immediately after the birth of a child until one month of age.

Neurogenic bladder   A condition in which there is an abnormality of the nerve supply to the lower urinary tract that results in either urinary incontinence or urinary retention (incomplete emptying of urine from the bladder) or both conditions.

Oncologist   A medical doctor who specializes in the treatment of cancer.

Ostium   A small opening in the abdomen that is connected to an organ such as the intestine or urinary tract. The ostium is surgically created to manage a difficult problem of eliminating stool or urine. See *stoma*.

Ostomy nurse   A specially trained nurse who is expert in all of the different kinds of problems that a person with an ostomy experiences.

Palpable   An adjective that refers to whether or not an abnormality can be palpated. For example, "the man had a *palpable* mass on his prostate."

Palpate   A medical term that means to feel with your hands and fingers. For example, "the doctor inserted his index finger into the rectum and *palpated* the prostate."

Paraplegia   A person who has both legs paralyzed but has the use of his or her arms and hands. Paraplegia results from spinal cord injury below the neck, usually in the thoracic or lumbar spinal region.

Pessary   An appliance, like a diaphragm, that is placed in the vagina to hold a prolapsed, or dropped, organ in place. It is usually shaped like a donut and comes in many different sizes.

Prolapse   A medical term that means to slide forward or downward. Genital prolapse refers to a falling down of the bladder, uterus, or rectum through the vagina. The medical term for prolapsed bladder is *cystocele*, and for prolapsed rectum, *rectocele.* Prolapsed uterus, which ought to be called uterocele, is called instead prolapsed uterus. Go figure!

Prompted voiding   A form of behavior modification. A voiding diary is kept for 24 hours by a caregiver and the time and amount of each urination and incontinent episode are recorded. With simple logic it is possible to plan the best times for the patient to urinate in order to stay dry. The caregiver then reminds or assists the patient to void at the designated time. Many patients regain full bladder control over the course of weeks or months when this technique is used.

PSA (Prostate-specific antigen)   A protein secreted by both normal and cancerous prostate tissue. In the bloodstream, some of the PSA is free and some is bound (attached) to proteins. Each can be measured separately and reported as total and free PSA. Just as the prostate grows with advancing age, so does the PSA increase with increasing age and prostate size. The relationship between age, prostate size, and PSA level is a complicated one, and many doctors believe that there are age-specific and size-specific normal values of PSA. However, PSA also rises as the prostate enlarges so there is no exact way to determine whether or not there is cancer by measuring PSA alone. Recently, it has been suggested that measurement of free PSA in the blood might be a more accurate way of screening for prostate cancer. The lower the free PSA, the greater the chances of prostate cancer. Men with less than 20–25% free PSA are thought to have the greatest chance of having prostate cancer.

PVR (Postvoid residual urine)   The amount of urine remaining in the bladder immediately after urinating.

Quadriplegia   Paralysis of all four extremities that results from injuries to the neck (cervical spine).

Radiation oncologist   A radiologist who specializes in the treatment of cancer using X-ray therapy.

Rectocele   A prolapse, or falling down, of the rectum through the vagina.

Regional anesthesia   Anesthesia of a certain region of the body usually achieved with either spinal or epidural injection of the anesthetic medication. You feel nothing once the anesthetic has taken effect. In addition, most people prefer also to receive a sedative, relaxant, or hypnotic medication, which puts them to sleep. If you prefer, though, you can remain wide awake.

Retrograde ejaculation   Backward flow of semen to the bladder instead of out the tip of the penis during ejaculation. This is not harmful, and you usually can't even feel the difference. The only negative effect is that it may be difficult or even impossible to father children.

Spincteric incontinence   Loss of urinary control due to malfunction of the urinary sphincter. It is like a leaky valve.

Saline   Salt water that mimics the chemical contents of body fluids.

SIC   Self intermittent catheterization.

Stoma   A surgically made opening in the abdomen that connects to the urinary tract. A continent stoma must be catheterized three to five times a day by the patient. An incontinent stoma requires the use of an appliance, which lies on the abdomen, attached to the stoma. Urine drains into the appliance, which is usually connected to a leg bag where the urine is stored. The leg bag is periodically emptied throughout the day.

Suprapubic catheter   An indwelling catheter that is placed directly into the bladder and comes out through a small opening in the lower abdomen. It may be placed under local anesthesia over a needle or it may be placed at the time of surgery. Indwelling catheters should be changed every two to four weeks.

Transitional cell epithelium   Cells that line the inside of the bladder and urethra. They give a similar appearance to the lining of the inside of the mouth.

Ureters   The tubes that carry urine from the kidney into the bladder.

Urethra   The tube that carries urine from the bladder out of the body during urination.

Urethrocele   A prolapse, or falling down, of the urethra through the vagina.

Urethrovaginal fistula   An abnormal opening that connects the urethra to the vagina. It is almost always the result of childbirth or surgery.

Urinary diversion   An operation that diverts urine from the bladder. It is performed by disconnecting the ureters from the bladder and connecting them to a segment of intestine that is attached to the skin, forming a stoma.

Urinary sphincter   A valvelike mechanism located in the wall of the urethra at its junction with the bladder. The purpose of the sphincter is to control the flow of urine. It is largely composed of muscles that stay closed and prevent urine leakage during the bladder filling and open to let the urine out during urination.

Urine culture   A test to determine whether or not there are any bacteria in the urine. It is performed by placing a drop of urine on a culture plate containing agar, a jellylike substance full of nutrients that promote the growth and multiplication of bacteria. If there are bacteria in the urine, they will start to grow and form colonies on the agar and, within a few days, they'll be visible to the naked eye. The type of bacteria can be determined by the color and appearance of the colonies. The number of bacteria are determined by estimating the number of colonies per milliliter. Most urinary tract infections have colony counts greater than

100,000 colonies per milliliter, but sometimes as little as 10,000 colonies per milliliter can cause infection.

Urodynamics   One or more of a series of tests that are designed to diagnose the cause of your bladder symptoms. A small catheter is passed through your urethra and into the bladder. Usually another catheter is passed into the rectum. The bladder is filled with fluid to simulate natural filling of urine from the kidneys. During bladder filling, you will be asked about your sensations and you'll be checked for incontinence. When you get the urge, you'll be asked to urinate. During this whole process, the pressure in the bladder and rectum are monitored and, in most instances, the exact cause of your symptoms can be determined.

Urologist   A physician and surgeon who specializes in disorders of the upper and lower urinary tract.

Vesicoureteral reflux   Backflow of urine from the bladder to the kidneys through the ureters. Normally, urine from the kidneys is transported to the bladder through two thin muscular tubes called ureters. Once it enters the bladder, urine is prevented from backing into the ureters because of the way in which the ureters enter the bladder and some other muscular properties of the bladder and ureters themselves.

Vesicovaginal fistula   An abnormal opening connecting the bladder with the vagina. It is almost always the result of childbirth or surgery.

Void   A synonym for urinate.

Appendix A:
Commonly Prescribed Medications

Medications can be purchased either in generic form or by brand name. Brand-name medications are manufactured by the company that did the research to develop the drug. The medication is in exactly the form that was originally approved by the FDA. A generic medication is required by law to contain the same active ingredients as its brand-name counterpart but may contain other (nonmedication) components that are different. For example, a generic medication may contain dyes to alter the color or sugar to alter the taste. The actual medication, though, must be identical with respect to the amount of drug, the dosage, and the form (pill, patch, liquid, or injection).

Brand-name drugs are usually more expensive than the generic preparation, in large part because of the extraordinary expense of complying with FDA regulations and doing the original research. The decision as to whether to purchase a generic or brand-name drug is not so simple. Some people think that brand-name drugs are better quality and undergo better quality control. Others disagree. Further, if we only pay for the generic medications, eventually there will be no financial incentive for pharmaceutical companies to develop new drugs.

Whenever a medication is prescribed for you, before you begin taking it, you should get answers to the following questions:

- Why are you taking the medication, i.e., what is it supposed to do?
- How often should you take it?
- When should you take it? With meals, after meals? With milk or water?

- Should you take it continuously or only when you have symptoms?
- When should you discontinue the medication?
- What are the expected and possible side effects?
- Which side effects are important to report to your doctor?
- Are there any side effects that constitute an emergency?
- Are there any restrictions that you should adhere to while taking it (alcohol, driving, sunlight, etc.)?
- Can the medication be taken with your other medications (including over-the-counter drugs)?
- Does the medication have any addictive properties?

Listed below are medications that are commonly used to treat people with lower urinary tract symptoms (LUTS) or medications that are used to treat other conditions, but have side effects that can cause LUTS. If you want to know more about the medications you are taking or if you develop new symptoms while on a medication, you should check with your doctor or pharmacist or read about it in one of the books listed in Appendix C.

The medications are listed in categories according to what they are intended to treat and how they are thought to work. Some of these medications, although FDA approved for other reasons, have never been FDA approved for treatment of urinary tract symptoms. Nevertheless, many have been shown to be both safe and effective and it is perfectly legal and appropriate for your doctor to prescribe them for these conditions if he thinks it necessary.

The generic names are listed first, followed by the brand-name drugs in parenthesis. If you have further questions, you should check with your doctor or pharmacist or look it up in one of the books listed in Appendix C.

WARNING: In this section, only the most common uses, side effects, and complications are listed. By necessity, the description of these medications is very incomplete. You should never take a prescription medication except with the advice and supervision of a health care provider licensed to prescribe medications.

Nocturia (urinating at night)

Antidiuretic hormone (ADH). Antidiuretic hormone is a substance produced by the pituitary gland in the brain. It signals the kidneys to cut back on urine production. It is normally secreted in response to dehydration. There is one synthetic product available:

Desmopressisn (DDAVP). For nocturia, only the nasal spray formulation is used. It has not been approved by the FDA for use in nocturia and should be used with caution in patients suspected of being prone to electrolyte abnormalities, those with heart failure, or those with disorders of thirst.

Prostatic Obstruction

Alpha-adrenergic blockers. Alpha-adrenergic blockers are medications that block the action of norepinephrine and cause relaxation of the smooth muscles of the prostatic urethra. The medications are given to reduce the muscular tone of the prostatic urethra and relieve prostatic obstruction. Common alpha-adrenergic blockers include:

Doxazosin (Cardura)
Prazosin (Minipres)
Phenoxybenzamine (Dibenzyline)
Terazosin (Hytrin)
Tamsulosin (Flowmax)

Common side effects include postural hypotension (a fall in blood pressure when changing from a lying down posture to a sitting or standing position), fatigue, diarrhea, dizziness, drowsiness, depression, fluid retention, nasal stuffiness, heart palpitations, and retrograde ejaculation.

It is recommended that all of these medications be taken at bedtime to minimize the possibility of side effects due to changes in position. Even when side effects occur, they often subside over time.

Phenoxybenzamine, in very large doses, has been shown to cause cancer in laboratory animals and it is recommended that it not be taken for a long time. There is no evidence that it causes cancer in humans, however.

5 alpha-reductase inhibitors. 5 alpha-reductase inhibitors are substances that block the conversion of the male hormone testosterone to dihydrotestosterone. Dihydrotestosterone is partially responsible for the growth of the prostate. Administration of 5 alpha-reductase inhibitors causes the prostate to shrink. The only FDA-approved 5 alpha-reductase inhibitor is:

Finasteride (Proscar)

Common side effects include diminished libido (sex drive), impotence, and a reduced volume of semen during ejaculation. These side effects are said to be completely reversible in most cases when the medication is discontinued.

It also causes the PSA (prostatic-specific antigen) blood level to fall by about 50%. It does not appear to decrease (or increase) the likelihood of developing prostate cancer, but the lowered PSA may make it more difficult to rely on PSA screening for early detection of prostate cancer.

Stress Incontinence

Alpha-adrenergic agonists. Alpha-adrenergic agonists are medications that mimic the action of norepinephrine, a neurotransmitter that stimulates the smooth muscle of the urethra to contract. These medications, which are given to people with incontinence due to sphincter weakness, help the sphincter stay closed and thereby improve continence. Common alpha-adrenergic agonists include:

Ephedrine sulfate (Sudafed)
Phenylpropanolamine hydrochloride (Ornade, Dexatrim)

These medications are usually prescribed for colds and allergies, but also for stress incontinence. They are the main ingredient in many over-the-counter nose drops, allergy and cold medications, and diet pills.

Common side effects: urethral obstruction, difficulty urinating, and even urinary retention. Accordingly, they should be used with caution in people with known urethral obstruction or a weak bladder. They also may cause rapid heartbeat, anxiety or nervousness, insomnia, or high blood pressure.

Common drug interactions: tricyclic antidepressants, antihypertensive medication.

Urinary Tract Pain

Urinary tract analgesics. Urinary tract analgesics are thought to have a specific pain-reducing effect on the urothelium (the mucosal lining of the bladder and urethra). The mechanism of action is not known, but they are often prescribed as an adjunct to antibiotics for cystitis and prostatitis and as treatment for other painful bladder and prostate conditions when infection is not present. Urinary tract analgesics include:

Phenazopyridine hydrochloride (Pyridium)
Phenazopyridine, hyoscyamine, butabarbital (Pyridiumn Plus)
Phenazopyridine hydrochloride plus sulfer antibiotic (Azo Gantrisin, Azo Gantanol)

Common side effects include orange-stained urine and nausea. More serious effects: jaundice, anemia.

Dimethyl sulfoxide (RIMSO-50). Also known as DMSO, this medication is a clear liquid that is instilled into the bladder through a catheter. It is thought to reduce pain that is coming from the bladder.

Common side effects: a garlic taste in the mouth usually occurs a few minutes after administration. Instillations are usually uncomfortable.

Sodium pentosan polysulfate (Elmiron). This medication was recently approved by the FDA for the treatment of interstitial cystitis. It is supplied as a capsule for oral ingestion to be taken at a dosage of 100 mg three times a day.

Urinary Tract Infections

There are two kinds of medications used to treat urinary tract infections—antibiotics and antibacterial/antiseptic agents, of which there are many different kinds. Only the most common side effects for the group as a whole are listed. For information on specific medications, you should consult your physician or pharmacist.

1. **Antibiotics.** Antibiotics are substances that are produced by a fungus, bacteria, or other organism that kill or inhibit the growth of microorganisms. Common side effects include loss of appetite, nausea, vomiting, stomach cramps, diarrhea, drowsiness, dizziness, headache, chills, fever, dry mouth, joint pain, minor allergic reactions, and vaginal yeast infections. More serious effects: severe allergic reaction (anaphylaxis).

   Aminoglycosides. These medications are used for serious or resistant urinary infections and are only administered by injection (intravenous or intramuscular).
   Gentamicin (Garamycin)
   Tobramycin (Tobramycin)
   Amikacin (Amikin)

   Serious side effects: temporary or permanent damage to hearing and to the kidneys. These complications are usually dose related (the longer the duration of treatment and the larger the dose, the greater the likelihood of developing the complication).

   Cephalosporins: Cephalosporins are antibiotics that are chemically related to penicillin. Approximately 10% of people who are allergic to penicillin are also allergic to cephalosporins. There are three categories of cephalosporins that correspond, in part, to the kinds of bacteria that they are effective against.

1st-generation cephalosporins:
  Cephazolin (Ancef, Kefzol)
  Cephalexin (Cephalexin, Keflex, Keftab)
2nd-generation cephalosporins:
  Cefaclor (Ceclor)
  Cefadroxil (Duricef)
  Cefuroxime (Ceftin)
  Cephradine (Cephradine)
3rd-generation cephalosporins:
  Ceftazidime (Fortaz, Tazicef, Tazidime)
  Ceftriaxone (Rocephin)

Fosfomycin. This is a new class of antibiotic.
Fosfomycin (Monurol). This is the only FDA-approved single-dose medication for the treatment of urinary tract infection. It is approved only for uncomplicated urinary tract infections.

Macrolides
Erythromycin (E-Mycin, Erythromycin). Erythromycin is not a first line antibiotic for urinary tract infections, but is sometimes used in patients who are allergic to penicillin and for patients with chlamydia trachomata infections.

Adverse drug interactions: Erythromycin can increase the effects of theophylline, an asthma medication, and cause serious, sometime fatal, complications. The E-Mycin brand of this drug is specially coated to lessen stomach irritation.

Penicillins (Amoxil, Augmentin, Bicillin, Geocillin, Mezlin, Omnipen, Pipracil, Spectrobid, Ticar, Unipen)

Quinolones
  Ciprofloxacin (Cipro)
  Cinoxacin (Cinobac)
  Levofloxacin (Levaquin)
  Lomefloxacin (Maxaquin)
  Nalidixic acid (NegGram)
  Norfloxacin (Noroxin)
  Ofloxacin (Floxin)

Drug interactions: Some of the quinolones increase the risk of drug overdose with theophylline, and should be used with extreme caution in patients who need to take theophylline.

Sulfonamides
Sulfamethoxazole (Bactrim, Gantanol, Septra)
Sulfisoxazole (Azo-Gantrisin, Gantrisin)

Tetracyclines
Doxycycline (Vibramycin)
Minocycline (Minocin)
Oxytetracycline (Terramycin)
Tetracycline (Achromycin)

Serious side effects: Tetracycline can interfere with bone growth and tooth enamel deposition in children and in the fetus. It also causes skin sensitivity to sunlight.

Trimethoprim (Proloprim, Trimpex). This is most often prescribed in a combination form with sulfonamides: *Trimethoprim/sulfamethoxazole* (Bactrim, Cotrim, Septra)

2. **Antibacterial/antiseptics.** Antibacterial and antiseptic agents, which are not derived from other living organisms, are substances that either kill or inhibit the growth of microorganisms.
Methenamine (Mandelamine)
Nitrofurantoin (Macrodantin, Macrobid, Nitrofurantoin)

Urinary Urgency and Urge Incontinence

Anticholinergic and antispasmodic medications. These medications block the effects of acetylcholine, a neurotransmitter that causes the bladder to contract, and/or have a direct relaxant effect on the smooth muscle of the bladder. They are given to stop the bladder from contracting involuntarily.

Flavoxate hydrocholride (Urispas)
Oxybutynin (Ditropan)
PropanthelineI (ProBanthine)
Dicyclomine (Bentyl)
Hyoscyamine (Cystospaz, Levsin, Anaspaz)

Hyoscyamine relaxes smooth muscles and inhibits spasms of the smooth muscle of the bladder and urethra. These drugs should not be taken by people with sensitivity to atropinelike drugs or those who have heart problems or glaucoma.

Side effects: drowsiness, dry mouth, skin sensitivity to sunlight, constipation, urinary retention.

More serious side effects: increased heart rate, dizziness, blurred vision or eye pain. *If these occur, the drug should be discontinued immediately and a physician notified.*

Urised. Urised is a combination of a urinary antiseptic (methenamine), atropine, and hyoscyamine. It also contains methylene blue, which will turn the urine blue or green, depending on how acid (blue) or alkaline (green) it is.

Serious side effects: severe dry mouth, rapid pulse, dizziness, blurred vision, and urinary retention. *If any of these effects occur, the drug should be discontinued immediately.*

Tricyclic antidepressants. These drugs have a sedative effect and may work by interfering with the activity of norepinephrine and serotonin, two substances that promote nerve activity. They may be used alone or in combinations with anticholinergic/antispasmodic agents. They may interact with a number of other medications, so it is particularly important that your doctor check the other medications you are taking to be sure that it is safe.

Amitriptyline (Amitrip, Elavil)
Desipramine (Norpramine)
Doxepin (Sinequan)
Imipramine (Tofranil)
Nortriptyline (Aventyl, Pamelor)
Protriptyline (Vivactil)
Trazadone (Desyrel)

Appendix B: Professional and Patient Advocacy Organizations

PROFESSIONAL ORGANIZATIONS

American Urologic Association, Inc.
1120 North Charles Street
Baltimore, MD 21201
Tel: 410-727-1100
Fax: 410-223-4370
E-mail: aua@auanet.org

American Foundation for Urologic
    Disease (AFUD)
1128 North Charles Street
Baltimore, MD 21201
410-468-1800
http://www.access.digex.net'afud
E-mail: admin@afud.org

American Board of Urology (ABU)
2216 Ivy Road, Suite 210
Charlottesville, VA 22903
Tel: 804-979-0059
Fax: 804-979-0266

International Continence Society
Bristol Urological Institute
Southmead Hospital
Bristol BS10 5NB, United Kingdom

Tel: 44(117)959-5690
Fax: 44(117)962-2970

Urodynamics Society
Division of Urology
University of Pennsylvania
    Medical Center
1st Floor Rhodes Pavilion
3400 Spruce Street
Philadelphia, PA 19104
Tel: 215-662-6755
Fax: 215-662-3955

American College of Obstetrics
    and Gynecology (ACOG)
409 12th St. South West
Washington, DC 20090
800-673-8444
www.acug.org

American Board of Obstetrics and
    Gynecology
2915 Vine Street
Dallas, TX 75204
214-871-1619

American Urogynecology Society
401 North Michigan Ave.
Chicago, IL 60611
312-644-6610

Society of Urologic Nurses and
Associates

East Holly Avenue—Box 56
Pitman, NJ 08071-0056
Tel: 609-256-2335
Fax: 609-589-7483
E-mail: sun@mail.ajj.com
http://www.inurse.com/SUNA

PATIENT ADVOCACY ORGANIZATIONS

U.S. Continence Organizations

The National Association for
    Continence
PO Box 8310
Spartanberg, SC 29305-8310
Tel: 864-579-7900
Fax: 864-579-7902
www.nafc.org

The Interstitial Cystitis Association
    (ICA)
PO Box 1533
Madison Square Station
New York, NY 10159

The Simon Foundation
Box 815
Wilmette, IL 60091
800-23-simon

The United Ostomy Association
36 Executive Park, Suite 120
Irvine, CA 92714
800-826-0826
PO Box 17864
Milwaukee, WI 53217
Tel: (1) 414-964-1799
Fax: (1) 414-964-7176
URL:
    http://www/execpc.com/iffgd

International Continence Organizations

Continence Worldwide
Contact: Dr. Peter Lim
c/o Division of Urology
Toa Payoh Hospital
Singapore 1129
Tel: (065)254.2155
Fax: (065)242.7149
e-mail: rani@technet.sg
http://www.continenceworldwide.
    com

Australia

Continence Foundation of
    Australia Ltd.
59 Victoria Parade, Collingwood,
Victoria 3066
Tel: (61) 3 416 0857
Fax: (61) 3 415 1016
Contacts: Dr. Richard Millard,
    President
Tony Walsh, Executive Director

Austria

Medizinische Gesellschaft fur
    Inkontinenzhilfe Osterreich
Speckbacherstrasse 1
A-6020 Innsbruck
Tel: (43) 512 58 37 03

Fax: (43) 512 58 9476
Contact: Professor Dr. H.
  Madersbacher

Canada

The Canadian Continence
  Foundation
PO Box 66524, Cavendish Mall,
Cote St Luc, Quebec H2W 3J6
Tel: (1) 514 932 3535
Fax: (1) 514 932 3533
Contact: Malvina Klag, Executive
  Director

Denmark

Dansk Inkontinensforening
(The Danish Association of
  Incontinent People)
Rathsacksvej 8, 1862 Frederiskberg
  C
Tel: (45) 3325 5121
Fax: (45) 3325 8695
Contact: Gunnar Lose, President

France

Association d'Aide aux Personnes
  Incontinentes
19 avenue des Messine, 75008 Paris
Tel: (33) 40 76 63 00
Contact: Michel Lemoine, Vice
  President

Germany

Gesellschaft fur Inkontinenzhilfe
  e.V. (GIH)
Geschaftsstelle,
Friedrich-Ebert-Strasse 124,
34119 Kassel
Tel: (49) 561 78 06 04
Fax: (49) 561 77 67 70
Contact: Frau Christ Thiel

Ireland

The Irish Continence Interest
  Group Continence Service,
Lurgan Health and Social Services
Sloan Street, Lurgan, Northern
  Ireland
Contact: Maire Doyle

Israel

The Centre for Continence in the
  Elderly
Rambam Medical Centre, POB-9602,
Haifa 31096
Tel: (972) 4854 2098
Fax: (972) 4854 2883
Contact: Dr. Ilan Gruenwald

Japan

Japan Continence Action Society
Continence Centre, 103 Jurihaimu,
4-2 Zenpukuzi 1-Chome,
  Suginami-Ku
Tokyo, 167
Tel: (81) 3 3301 3860
Fax: (81) 3 3301 3587
Contact: Kaoru Nishimua

Netherlands

Stichting Incontinentie Nederland
University Hospital Maastricht,
Department of Urology, PO Box
  5800,
6202 AZ Maastricht
Tel: (31) 43 387 7258
Fax: (31) 43 387 5259
also at:
Muntelbolwerk 1, 5213 SZ Den
  Bosch
Tel: (31) 73 122 822
Fax: (31) 73 123 721
Contact: Professor R. A. Janknegt,
  Chairman

Vereniging Nederlandse
  Incontinentie Verpleekundigen
  (VNIV)
Kastanjestraat 21, 3434, CA
  Nieuwegein
Tel: (31) 30 606 0053
Fax: (31) 30 608 1312
Contact: Ulli Haase, Chairman

New Zealand

New Zealand Continence
  Association Inc.
41 Pembroke Street, Hamilton
Tel: (64) 7 834 3528
Fax: (64) 7 834 3532
E-mail: stuartb@wave.co.nz
Contact: Jill Brown, Secretary

Singapore

Society for Continence (Singapore)
c/o Division of Urology, Toa Payoh
  Hospital,
Tao Payoh Rise, Singapore 1129
Tel: (65) 254 2155/350 7558
Fax: (65) 251 9454/252 7149
Contacts: Dr. Peter Lim Huat Chye,
  President
Rani Vadiveloo, Executive Director

Slovenia

INKO, Slovensko Druotvo Za Pomo
Inkontinentnim Osebam
Stozice 23/B, 61113 Ljubljana
Tel/Fax: 611 168 5050
Contact: Marja Kop, Secretary

Sweden

Swedish Urotherapists
Nordenskioldsgatan 10
S-413 09, Goteborg
Tel: (46) 31 50 26 39
Fax: (46) 31 53 68 32
Contact: Brigitta Lindehall

United Kingdom

Association for Continence Advice
  (ACA)
Winchester House, Kensington
  Park,
Cranmer Road, London SW9 6EJ
Tel: (44) 171 820 8113
Fax: (44) 171 820 0442
Contact: Martin Eede, Executive
  Director

The Continence Foundation
2 Doughty Street, London WC1N
  2PH
Tel: (44) 171 404 6875
Fax: (44) 171 404 6876
URL: http://www.vois.org.uk/cf
Contact: David Pollock, Director

Enuresis Resource and Information
  Centre (ERIC)
34 Old School House, Britannia
  Road,
Kingswood, Bristol BS15 2DB
Tel: (44) 117 960 3060
Fax: (44) 117 960 0401
E-mail:
  106142.1477@compuserve.com
Contact: Penny Dobson, Director

inconTact
2 Doughty Street, London WC1N
  2PH
Fax: (44) 171 404 6876

Royal College of Nursing
  Continence Care Forum
c/o Royal College of Nursing
20 Cavendish Square, London
  WIM OAB
Tel: (44) 171 409 3333
Contacts: Angela Billington,
  Chairman
Sue Thomas, Community Advisor

OTHER PATIENT ADVOCACY ORGANIZATIONS

Eastern Paralyzed Veterans
   Association
75-20 Astoria Boulevard
Jackson Heights, NY 11370-1177
718-803-3782
www.epva.org.
E-mail: info@epva.org

National Spinal Cord Injury
   Hotline
2200 Kernan Drive
Baltimore, MD 21207
800-526-3456
http://users.aol.com-scihotline
E-mail: scihotline@aol.com

National Multiple Sclerosis Society
733 3rd Avenue
New York, NY 10017 3288
800-fight-ms
http://www.nmss.org

Parkinson's Disease Foundation
710 West 168th Street
New York, NY 10032
212-923-4700
http://www.parkinsons-
   foundation.org

American Diabetes Association
1660 Duke Street
Alexandria, VA 22314
800-DIABETES
www.diabetes.org

Spina Bifida Association of
   America
4590 MacArthur Blvd., NW, Suite
   250
Washington, DC 20007
800-621-3141
http://www.sbaa.org

National Stroke Association
8480 E. Orchard Road, Suite 1000
Englewood, CO 80111
303 771-1700

Brain Injury Association of New
   York State
10 Colvin Avenue
Albany, NY 12207
800-228-8201

Appendix C:
Other Reading Material

Burgio, K. L., Pearce, K. L., & Lucco, A. J., *Staying Dry*, The Johns Hopkins University Press, Baltimore, 1989.

Chalker, R., & Whitmore, K. E., *Overcoming Bladder Disorders*, Harper and Row, New York, 1990.

Gartley, C. B., *Managing Incontinence*, Jameson Books, Ottawa, Ill., 1985.

Kilmartin, A., *Understanding Cystitis*, Warner Books, New York, 1986.

Rybacki, J. J., & Long, J. W., *The Essential Guide to Prescription Drugs*, Harper Collins, New York, 1996.

Silverman, H. M., *The Pill Book*, Bantam Books, New York, 1996.

Smith, W., *Overcoming Cystitis: A Practical Self-Help Guide for Women*, Bantam Books, New York, 1987.

Walsh, P. C., & Worthington, J. F., *The Prostate: A Guide for Men and the Women Who Love Them*, The Johns Hopkins University Press, Baltimore, 1995.

Urinary Incontinence in Adults
Guide for Patients
AHCRP Publication Clearing
   House
PO Box 8547
Silver Spring, MD 20907-8547
800-358-9295
http://www.ahcpr.gov

Benign Prostatic Hyperplasia:
   Diagnosis and Treatment
Guide for Patients
AHCRP Publications Clearing
   House
PO Box 8547
Silver Spring, MD 20907-8547
800-358-9295
http://www.ahcpr.gov

The Surgical Management of Female
Stress Urinary Incontinence
Female Stress Urinary
    Incontinence Guidelines Panel
A Doctor's Guide for Patients
American Urological Association,
    Inc.

Health Policy Department
1120 N. Charles Street
Baltimore, MD 21201
410-223-4367
http://www.auanet.org

Index

Page numbers in *italics* indicate Glossary entries.

0528

0528